COLOUR GUIDE

Common Conditions

Michael G. Mead BSc MB BS DCH DRCOG MRCGP
General Practitioner, Leicester, UK

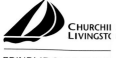

CHURCHILL
LIVINGSTONE

EDINBURGH LONDO ... ORONTO
1999

D1419067

CHURCHILL LIVINGSTONE
An imprint of Harcourt Brace and Company
Limited

© Harcourt Brace & Company Limited 1999

🖢 is a registered trade mark of Harcourt Brace
and Company Limited

The right of Michael G. Mead to be identified as
author of this work has been asserted by him in
accordance with the Copyright, Designs and
Patents Act 1988.

First published 1999

ISBN 0 443 06021 5

British Library Cataloguing in Publication Data
A catalogue record for this book is available from
the British Library.

Library of Congress Cataloging in Publication Data
A catalog record for this book is available from
the Library of Congress.

Medical knowledge is constantly
changing. As new information
becomes available, changes in
treatment, procedures, equipment
and the use of drugs become
necessary. The author and the
publishers have, as far as it is
possible, taken care to ensure
that the information given in this
text is accurate and up to date.
However, readers are strongly
advised to confirm that the
information, especially with
regard to drug usage, complies
with current legislation and
standards of practice.

The
publisher's
policy is to use
**paper manufactured
from sustainable forests**

Printed in China.
SWTC/01

For Churchill Livingstone

Publisher: Timothy Horne
Project Editor: Janice Urquhart
Copy Editor: Adam Campbell
Indexer: Helen McKillop
Design Direction: Erik Bigland
Project Controller: Frances Affleck

Preface and Acknowledgements

This book covers sixty of the commonest conditions suffered by humanity worldwide. Each chapter provides up-to-date, structured information on diagnosis, investigation and management. *Common Conditions* is therefore an invaluable tool for all workers in the health industry, and, in fact, anyone with an interest in medicine.

I would like to thank Practice Nurse and all those at Reed Healthcare Communications for permission to use some of the material originally published in the Common Conditions series featured in Practice Nurse in 1996/7.

I am indebted to the following for providing and helping with the photographs: consultants at the Leicester Royal Infirmary—Farook Al Azzawi (gynaecology), Kim Bibby (ophthalmology), Jim Cook (ENT), Dr A. Fletcher (pathology), David Ireland (gynaecology), Kim Krarup (radiology), Mark Lawden (neurology), George Murty (ENT), Ross Naylor (vascular surgery), Roger Oldham (rheumatology), Barrie Rathbone (gastroenterology), Ash Samanta (rheumatology) and Dr Iain Squire in the Department of Medicine; consultants at Glenfield General Hospital—Bob Bing (medicine), John de Caestecker (gastroenterology), Tony Gerschlick (cardiology), Richard Power (orthopaedics), David Rew (surgery), Adam Scott (surgery), Graham Taylor (orthopaedics) and Mr D. D. Vara of the respiratory Function Laboratory; consultants at Leicester General Hospital— Felix Burden (diabetes), Ashley Dennison (surgery), Steve Godsiff (orthopaedics), David Osborn (urology); consultant dermatologist, Walsgrave Hospital, Dr Berth-Jones; Schering Health Care Ltd for the photographs of the oestrogen patch and the Mirena intrauterine system and Merck, Sharp and Dohme for the illustration of the prostate gland.

Finally I would like to thank my ever tolerant patients, staff and partners.

The following Figures are reproduced with permission and remain the copyright of the Leicester Royal Infirmary: Figs 21, 22, 25–27, 31, 41, 42, 47, 48, 55, 56, 59–63, 71, 72, 76A & B, 77, 79, 80, 86, 91–93, 103, 107, 109–112, 126, 129, 130, 135, 136, 152–155, 160, 164, 166. Figure 128 reproduced with permission from Churchill Livingstone.

Contents

Prevalence and clinical features

Acne affects 85% of adolescents. Peak incidence is at age 19 and it usually lasts 10 years. Lesions are comedones (blackheads), inflammatory papules, pustules, cysts and nodules. The face, back and chest are affected (Figs 1–3); may scar. Distinguish from rosacea—erythema, pustules, papules after age 30, only on the face, usually in women.

Management

Advice. No evidence for diet; sunlight helps (but some treatments photosensitise); do not pick lesions; wash twice a day; use light non-greasy cosmetics; treat dandruff.

Topical therapy. For mild acne: need at least 8 weeks' therapy to assess benefit. Options: (1) Benzoyl peroxide—start with 5% daily for a few hours, increasing slowly to 10% if needed; mild erythema/peeling commonly occurs. (2) Topical retinoids—more effective for comedones; side-effect is skin irritation. Avoid in pregnancy. (3) Topical antibiotics twice daily. Antibiotic resistance is reduced by combining with benzoyl peroxide. (4) Azelaic acid—less irritating than benzoyl peroxide but there is a 6-month limit to treatment.

Systemic antibiotics. For moderate acne, e.g. oxytetracycline (not in pregnancy/children), erythromycin, minocycline, doxycycline. Try for 3 months, then reassess—should have improved but usually need at least 6 months, possibly 12. If the patient is on the contraceptive pill, advise extra contraception for at least the first 4 weeks of oral antibiotic use.

Hormonal therapy. For women with pill containing ethinyloestradiol 35 μg and cyproterone acetate 2 mg. Also contraceptive.

Nodulocystic/severe acne. Refer to dermatologist for treatment with isotretinoin. It is teratogenic and requires monitoring of lipids and liver function.

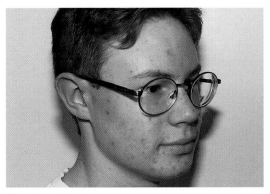

Fig. 1 Acne of the face.

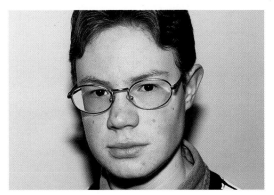

Fig. 2 Patient in Fig. 1 substantially improved after 4 months of oral antibiotics.

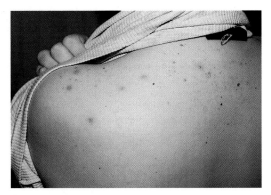

Fig. 3 Acne of the back.

2 / Alcoholism

Definition

Alcohol intake interfering significantly with a patient's social and physical functioning. Alcohol is measured in units (Fig. 4). Safe alcohol limits: women, 14 units/week; men, 21 units/week.

Clinical presentations

Physical: gastritis, peptic ulcers, obesity, pancreatitis, neuropathy, myopathy, hypertension, cardiac problems, fits, sexual dysfunction. Less than a third develop cirrhosis (Fig. 5), which can lead to liver failure, ascites, portal hypertension (associated with varices, which may cause severe upper GI tract bleeding; Fig. 6). Commonest physical presentations are nausea, anorexia, vomiting, tremor, repeated infections.
Mental: depression, anxiety, dementia, hallucinations, suicide.
Social: divorce, child abuse, violence, debt.
Legal/employment: crime, sickness absence, accidents, unemployment. Questionaires used in screening, e.g. CAGE questionnaire. Blood tests used: (1) full blood count—macrocytosis associated with alcoholism; (2) the gamma glutamyl transpeptidase (GGT)—raised in >80% of alcohol abusers. (Normal within 3 weeks of abstinence.)

Management

(1) Recognise by remembering 'at risk' situations. (2) Analyse quantity, pattern and reasons for drinking. (3) Explain risks and get patient to accept the problem. (4) Involve family and friends in support. (5) Advise patients on a strategy to combat their problem, using drink diaries, self-help packs, setting goals/targets. (6) Help with specific physical, financial, marital or social problems. (7) Maintain motivation by regular follow-up. (8) Refer to specialists if severe alcoholism is unresponsive to your efforts, there is major physical/psychiatric disease, severe withdrawal problems, no support available. (9) Detoxification with benzodiazepines/chlormethiazole is only required by a minority and needs close supervision. (10) Vitamin supplements if chronic problem/poor nutrition. (11) Specialist advice if using disulfiram or acamprosate for withdrawal.

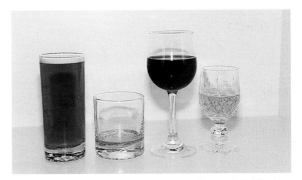

Fig. 4 Each glass contains a unit of alcohol—half a pint (284 mL) of beer (3.5% alcohol by volume, ABV), a single measure (25 mL) of spirits (40% ABV), a small glass (125 mL) of wine (8% ABV), and a small glass (50 mL) of sherry (20% ABV).

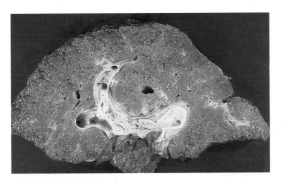

Fig. 5 The liver in a patient with cirrhosis.

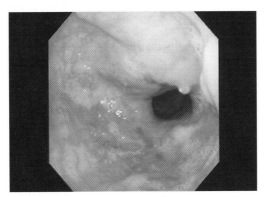

Fig. 6 Oesophageal varices at endoscopy. One has a white fibrin plug indicating recent bleeding.

3 / Anaemia

Definition and common causes

Haemoglobin <11.5 g/dL in females, <13.5 g/dL in males. Anaemia is microcytic if the mean corpuscular volume is <80 fL, macrocytic if >95 fL, normocytic if 80–95 fL, and hypochromic if mean corpuscular haemoglobin (MCH) is <27 pg.

Common causes of microcytic anaemia are iron deficiency and thalassaemia. Macrocytic anaemia associated with B_{12} or folate deficiency, liver disease and hypothyroidism. Normocytic anaemia occurs with chronic diseases, malignancies, renal failure and haemolysis (can also be macrocytic).

Clinical features

Symptoms depend on how quickly anaemia develops. May be asymptomatic until haemoglobin $<$ about 9 g/dL. Symptoms are pallor, tiredness, tachycardia, breathlessness on exertion, headache, giddiness/dizziness, tinnitus, anorexia, nausea, paraesthesiae. On examination, check mucous membranes for pallor, tongue for glossitis (in B_{12} deficiency), mouth for angular stomatitis and nails for koilonychia (iron deficiency). A full blood count (Fig. 7) will confirm anaemia.

Management

Find cause. Look at MCV, MCH. Iron deficiency anaemia is microcytic, hypochromic (Fig. 8)—confirm by serum iron and ferritin. Then investigate the cause of iron deficiency, e.g. blood loss (GI tract, menorrhagia), malabsorption, diet. If macrocytic, test B_{12}/folate and consider malabsorption and pernicious anaemia (confirmed by autoantibodies to parietal cells/intrinsic factor, megaloblasts in bone marrow).

If haemoglobin is very low and patient symptomatic, may need transfusion. If not, can replace iron orally (has GI side-effects, turns stools black) or by i.m. injection. Treatment of pernicious anaemia: i.m. hydroxocobalamin, alternate days for 10 days, then a 3-monthly maintenance dose.

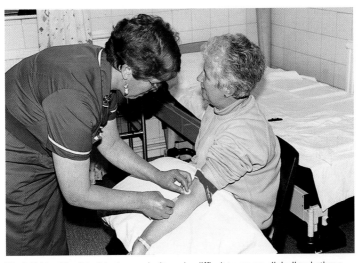

Fig. 7 Taking blood to detect anaemia: it can be difficult to assess clinically whether a patient with pallor has anaemia and how anaemic they might be.

Differential	Neutrophils	Lymphocytes	Monocytes	Eosinophils	Basophils	Atypical lymph.	Metamyelos.	Myelocytes
WBC %	68.5	23.8	6.0	0.7	1.0			
x 10⁷/l	2.81	0.98	0.25	0.03	0.04			
% Adult Normal Range ABS	40-75 2.0-7.5	20-45 1.5-4.0	2-10 0.2-0.8	1-6 0.04-0.4	1 or less 0.01-0.1			

Machine Differential	Granulocytes	Lymphocytes	Monocytes	WHITE CELL COMMENT
WBC %				
	%	%	%	

HYPOCHROMIC +++ MICROCYTIC +++ EXCLUDE Fe DEFICIENCY

> FILE
> NORMAL
> APPOINTMENT
> PRESCRIPTION
> NOTES PLEASE
> OTHER

*** URGENT REQUEST ***QUOTED NORMAL RANGES ARE FOR ADULTS

Hb M 13.5-18.0 F 11.5-16.5	RBC M 4.5-6.5 F 3.9-5.6	HCT M 0.4-0.54 F 0.37-0.47	MCV 80-99	MCH 27-32	Reticulocytes 0-2	WBC 4-11	Platelets 150-400	P.V. 1.5-1.7:
*5.0	*3.68	*0.199	*54.1	*13.6		4.1	*443	
g/dl	x 10¹²/l		fl	pg	%	x 10⁹/l	x 10⁹/l	cp

Fig. 8 The different measurements made on a full blood count can provide a clue to the underlying cause of the anaemia.

4 / Angina and myocardial infarction

Angina

Definition/clinical features

Chest pain/discomfort which is (1) central/ retrosternal but may radiate to arms, neck, throat, teeth, jaw; (2) 'tight', 'heavy', 'crushing'; (3) precipitated by exertion, relieved by rest or within 5–10 min of glyceryl trinitrate (GTN). Commonest cause is coronary artery disease.

Patient assessment

(1) Exclude other diagnoses, e.g. oesophagitis/ muscular. (2) Identify other causes (anaemia, aortic stenosis). (3) Examine pulse, BP, heart sounds, peripheral pulses. (4) Investigate: full blood count, urine, serum lipids, blood glucose, resting ECG (normal in >50%), thyroid function. Exercise ECG confirms ischaemia. (5) Advise on smoking, hyperlipidaemia, hypertension, diabetes, obesity, diet, exercise, alcohol.

Principles of management/ referral

(1) Refer—admit to hospital unstable angina (rapidly worsening angina/angina at rest for >15 min) after giving 300 mg aspirin; routine referral for diagnosis/assessment, complications, murmurs, post-infarction, poor control. (2) Advise on driving, work. (3) Reduce BP to <160/85, total cholesterol to <5.2 mmol/L (LDL cholesterol <3.4 mmol/L). (4) Treat—aspirin 150 mg/day plus GTN. If required, regular beta-blocker (if contraindicated diltiazem or verapamil). If uncontrolled on beta-blocker, add long-acting nitrate/calcium antagonist/potassium channel activator. May need surgery (angioplasty or coronary artery bypass graft, Figs 9 & 10).

Myocardial infarction

Severe chest pain >30 min. Diagnosed by ECG (Fig. 11) and cardiac enzymes. Immediate: aspirin 150 mg, i.v. diamorphine, thrombolytic treatment ideally within 90 min. Post-MI: rehabilitate, treat risk factors, lower total cholesterol to <4.8 mmol/L (LDL <3.2 mmol/L), aspirin 75–150 mg, beta-blockers, ACE inhibitors if patient develops heart failure/left ventricular dysfunction.

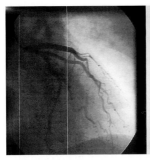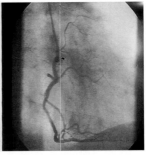

Fig. 9 Angiogram showing a block of the left anterior descending artery.

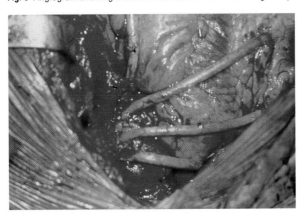

Fig. 10 Coronary artery bypass grafts.

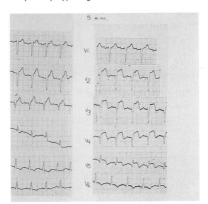

Fig. 11 ECG of an anterior myocardial infarction—note the ST elevation starting in the V₂ lead.

5 / Anxiety

Definition

Anxiety is a normal reaction to stress but a clinical disorder when symptoms are too severe, prolonged or occur without, or out of proportion to, a stressful event. It is a common feature in consultations (Fig. 12) and classified into groups—social phobia, panic disorder, post-traumatic stress etc.

Assessment of patient

(1) Identify anxiety—patients may present with poor concentration, fatigue, restlessness, irritability, anorexia, insomnia, tremor, palpitations, nausea, hyperventilation, sweating, headaches, giddiness, diarrhoea, muscle tension, paraesthesiae, multiple consultations for minor illness. (2) Take a history—symptom review, life events, fears, phobias, panic attacks, past medical history, family history, drug/alcohol misuse. (3) Exclude physical illness, e.g. thyrotoxicosis. (4) Differentiate from depression (depression suggested by early morning waking, guilt, hopelessness, weight loss, suicidal thoughts).

Management

(1) Reassure and allow patient time to talk. (2) Offer support and counselling. (3) Special psychological techniques to help specific patients—cognitive therapy, psychotherapy techniques, assertiveness training, relaxation techniques, distraction, exposure therapy for phobic patients, hypnosis. (4) Consider drug therapy. Beta-blockers reduce somatic symptoms. If mixed anxiety and depression, treat with an antidepressant. Use benzodiazepines short-term (2–4 weeks); warn patients re. driving/effect on judgement. Dependence can occur in 4 weeks—withdraw patients slowly, first changing to a long-acting one, e.g. diazepam. Buspirone is an anxiolytic that is slower in action than benzodiazepines but without the dependence/withdrawal problems. (5) Referral to psychiatrist/psychologist for patients with specific anxiety disorders/severe symptoms unresponsive to treatment and for special psychological techniques.

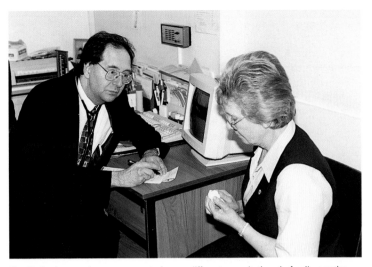

Fig. 12 Anxiety can be a component of many different consultations in family practice.

Cause of abdominal pain

Common causes of abdo pain are anxiety, gastroenteritis/gastritis, dietary indiscretion, constipation. Other causes include: appendicitis, renal/biliary colic, peptic ulceration, diverticulitis, pancreatitis, peritonitis, gynaecological causes.

Diagnosis

History. Include site, character, radiation of pain, associated features, last menstrual period. Appendicitis is classically central abdominal pain moving to the right iliac fossa after a few hours and associated with anorexia, nausea and vomiting. In children this history is unusual; consider appendicitis in any ill child with abdo pain and/or vomiting.

Examination. Include position/posture (still/rolling in agony with colic), measuring temperature, palpating abdomen, testes and hernial orifices, performing a rectal examination. Classically, appendicitis presents with a mild fever, tenderness in the right iliac fossa and tenderness on the right side with rectal examination. An abnormal appendix position gives different symptoms/signs, e.g. pelvic appendicitis may cause diarrhoea/ urinary symptoms and be detected only on rectal examination. Main differential diagnosis of appendicitis is mesenteric adenitis in children, gynaecological/urinary problems in young females. Crohn's disease (Fig. 13) can present with acute abdo pain resembling appendicitis.

Tests. Urine for infection, sugar and blood. Full blood count may show a raised white count in appendicitis.

Follow-up. If in doubt, arrange a repeat consultation/visit. As a general rule a patient with abdo pain lasting >6h is likely to need hospital admission.

Management

Depends on diagnosis. If suspected appendicitis, admit to hospital urgently for appendicectomy (Fig. 14; scar of appendicectomy in right iliac fossa, Fig. 15).

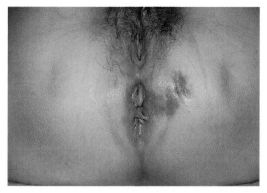

Fig. 13 Crohn's disease; in this case there are skin tags around the anus and a red area of induration on the left buttock due to previous fistulae and sepsis.

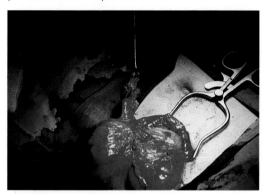

Fig. 14 Removing the appendix.

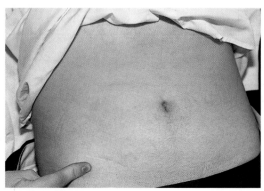

Fig. 15 Scar of appendicectomy.

7 / Asthma

An inflammatory disease with reversible airways narrowing—the airways have increased responsiveness to many factors, e.g. treatment.

Common presentations

Recurrent or exercise-induced cough/wheeze/ breathlessness. Remember recurrent cough, especially nocturnal, in children.

Diagnosis

(1) Take history—personal/family history of asthma, eczema, allergic rhinitis, urticaria, relation of symptoms to exercise, precipitating factors, diurnal variation. (2) Examine chest. (3) Demonstrate airways variability by peak expiratory flow rates (PEFRs, Fig. 16)—reversibility test: ≥15% rise in PEFR 5–10 min after two puffs of bronchodilator; exercise test: fall in PEFR ≥15% within 10 min of exercise; diurnal variation: ≥15% diurnal PEFR variation. May need oral steroid trial.

Management

(1) Patient education—stop smoking, avoid allergens, use self-management plans. (2) Drugs— early use of anti-inflammatories. (3) Follow-up— compliance, symptoms, PEFRs, device selection, inhaler technique (Fig. 17).

Acute

Oxygen, bronchodilator, steroids. Measure PEFR, heart rate, respiration to assess severity.

Chronic

Use British Thoracic Society guidelines. For chronic asthma in adults and schoolchildren:
   Step 1—occasional use of short-acting beta-agonist bronchodilator. Step 2—add regular inhaled anti-inflammatory: steroid or cromoglycate/nedocromil. Step 3—use short-acting beta-agonist plus high-dose inhaled steroid or low-dose inhaled steroid plus long-acting inhaled beta-agonist. Step 4—high-dose inhaled steroids (use spacers, Fig. 18), regular bronchodilators plus trial of inhaled long-acting beta-agonist or theophyllines or inhaled ipratropium, etc. Step 5— add regular steroid tablets.
   Steps for children <5. 1: bronchodilator; 2: adds inhaled cromoglycate or inhaled steroid; 3: increases dose of inhaled steroid; 4: high-dose inhaled steroids plus bronchodilator.

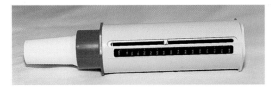

Fig. 16 A peak flow meter: patients with asthma should monitor their readings.

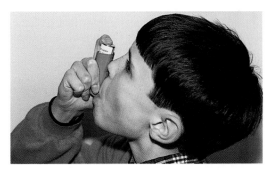

Fig. 17 A child using an inhaler: teaching inhaler technique is very important.

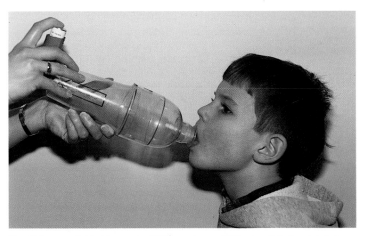

Fig. 18 A spacer is ideal for use in children and essential if using high-dose inhaled steroids.

8 / Backache

Causes

About 80% have mechanical/ligamentous backache; up to 20% a prolapsed intervertebral disc (PID); in a minority a disease is the cause.

Diagnosis

History. Mechanical backache worse on movement; relieved by rest; locally tender. A PID may have shooting (sciatic) pain radiating down leg with numbness/weakness/paraesthesiae. Beware a central disc prolapse with severe leg weakness, saddle area anaesthesia and urinary symptoms/retention. Suggesting an underlying disease are: severe, worsening pain; night pain; morning stiffness; weight loss; age >50 or <20.

Examination. Look for curvature of spine (Fig. 19), local tenderness, limitation of movement, straight leg raising (with PID, Fig. 20). Further examination (leg reflexes, sensation) depends on symptoms.

Tests. Plain X-ray unhelpful unless disease or structural abnormality like spondylolisthesis (Fig. 21) suspected. ESR/plasma viscosity and alkaline phosphatase are the most useful blood tests. MRI scan can help diagnose PID.

Management

Central disc prolapse. Requires emergency admission.

Mechanical backache. Advise to avoid bed rest, maintain normal activities, take regular analgesia. Educate re. back care; manipulate if pain does not settle in a few days. If no return to work/activity within 6 weeks, recommend and start back exercises (physiotherapist/osteopath/chiropractor).
PID with nerve root pain. May need bed rest, analgesia, muscle relaxant but avoid prolonged bed rest; mobilise as soon as possible. An epidural may help recovery. Most recover in 4–6 weeks. Those who do not, or develop progressive leg weakness, need urgent referral. Options then include shrinking the disc by injecting chymopapain (chemonucleolysis) or surgical discectomy.
Backache due to a disease process. Needs referral, e.g. ankylosing spondylitis (Fig. 22).

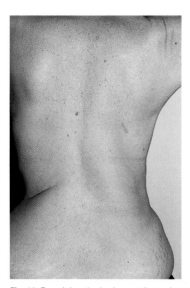

Fig. 19 Examining the back may give a clue to the cause—this patient has a scoliosis.

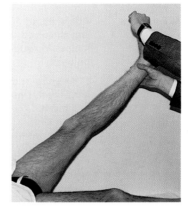

Fig. 20 Testing straight leg raising—limitation suggests a prolapsed intervertebral disc.

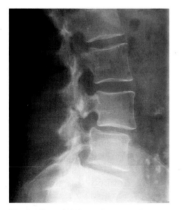

Fig. 21 Spondylolisthesis—note the forward shift of one vertebra on another.

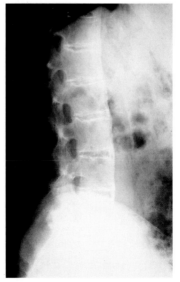

Fig. 22 Ankylosing spondylitis, showing the classical 'bamboo spine' with calcification of the intervertebral ligaments.

9 / Bed-wetting (nocturnal enuresis)

Prevalence	About 5% of 10-year-olds and 15% of 5-year-olds wet their bed at least once a week. Contributing factors include family history, stress and nocturnal polyuria.
Causes	(1) Primary monosymptomatic nocturnal enuresis (PNE) with positive family history and no daytime symptoms. (2) Secondary nocturnal enuresis where bed-wetting occurs after at least 6 months' dryness—associated with stress, urinary tract infection (UTI). (3) Detrusor instability where there may be frequency, urgency, urge incontinence. (4) UTI. (5) Anatomical abnormalities, e.g. ectopic ureter. (6) Diabetes mellitus and renal failure.
Diagnosis	*History.* Family history, urinary symptoms (stream, frequency, urgency, dribbling), secondary bed-wetting after dry period, pattern of bed-wetting (frequency, quantity, daytime wetting), bowel problems/soiling, stress, family's reaction and management.
	Examination. Include plotting on growth chart, abdomen (including bladder), genitalia and lower limbs. Record blood pressure, test urine for sugar/protein and exclude a UTI.
Management	Treat specific pathology (investigate if UTI); usually none found. No treatment recommended below age 5. Treat soiling before bed-wetting.
	(1) Advice—reassurance, encourage parental tolerance, toilet child before bedtime, use a waterproof mattress cover. No need to restrict fluids. (2) Star chart (Fig. 23) with rewards helpful, especially if aged 5–7. (3) Enuresis alarm (Fig. 24) useful after age 7. Helps about two-thirds of children; more if combined with 'dry bed training'—a special waking regime. (4) Drugs—tricyclics rarely used (side-effects, overdose risk). Try desmopressin nasal spray/tablets for children over age 5, initially for 3 months—effective, but high relapse rate on stopping the drug.

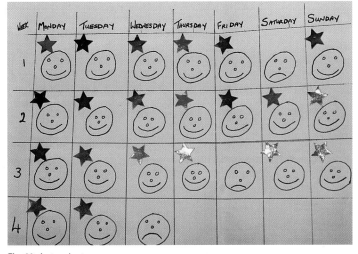

Fig. 23 A star chart.

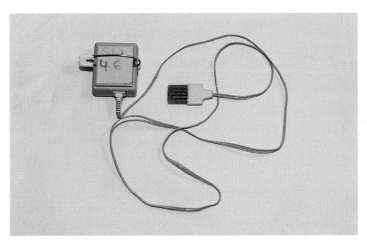

Fig. 24 An enuresis alarm.

Cause

Benign breast disorders include cysts, fibroadenomas, duct ectasia, areas of nodularity, hyperplasia. Breast cancer incidence increases with age.

Patient assessment

Take a history—size, duration, relation to period, associated symptoms, use of pill/HRT, past history of breast problems, family history of breast cancer. (2) Examine—four breast quadrants, axillae and supraclavicular fossae. Suggesting cancer are: nipple changes (including retraction), irregularity, hardness, skin tethering, immobility, palpable nodes, skin oedema/dimpling. Age >35 is a risk factor. Note that breast pain/nipple discharge rarely due to cancer.

Management

No lump found. Re-examine after a period. Teach breast self-examination.

Lump palpable. Breast cyst in younger patient: aspirate (Figs 25–27) and review in 2–3 weeks. If cyst still palpable or blood-stained fluid, refer. Younger patients (< age 25) with small (<2 cm) lump with benign features: fine-needle aspiration for cytology and review. Refer all other lumps to a breast specialist for fine-needle aspiration and ultrasound (≤ age 35) or fine-needle aspiration and mammography (> age 35). Refer a patient with a nipple discharge and lump. Cyclical breast pain and no specific lump may respond to gamolenic acid or danazol.

Standard treatment of breast cancer is wide local excision of lump and axillary dissection of nodes plus radiotherapy, but depends on tumour; chemotherapy is also used. Tamoxifen prevents relapses and improves survival but there is an increased risk of endometrial carcinoma with long-term use.

Screening using mammography

In the UK the breast screening programme is 3-yearly in women aged 50–64 by mammography; 2-yearly screening would improve the pick-up rate.

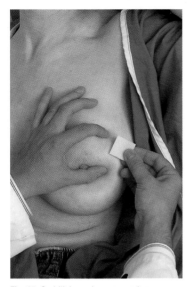

Fig. 25 Stabilising a breast cyst between the fingers.

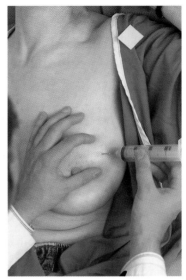

Fig. 26 Inserting the needle.

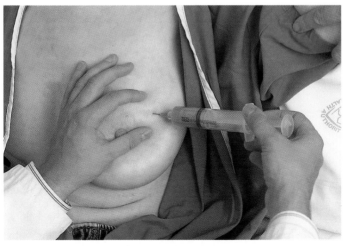

Fig. 27 Aspirating the cyst.

Cataracts

A cataract (Fig. 28) is a lens opacity, impairing vision in 40% of the over-75s. Causes include ageing, diabetes, congenital, trauma, uveitis, steroid therapy. Patient presents with visual loss, possibly with visual blurring. Light may be scattered or dazzle, making night driving difficult. Diagnosis confirmed by ophthalmoscopy. Test vision using a Snellen chart. Exclude other eye disease—may need to refer for this.

Treatment Day case surgery with either extracapsular extraction of the lens or phacoemulsification, replacing with an artificial lens.

Glaucoma

Commonest form is open-angle glaucoma. A blinding disease characterised by raised intraocular pressure (IOP >21mmHg), cupped optic discs (Fig. 29) and visual field loss. Patients with raised IOPs without optic nerve damage/visual field loss have ocular hypertension and are at risk of glaucoma. A low tension glaucoma also exists, with normal IOP but optic nerve damage/visual field loss. Symptoms include blurred vision and haloes around lights, but may not be detected until significant visual loss has occurred. Acute closed-angle glaucoma presents with a painful red eye, vision grossly reduced and a dilated fixed pupil.

Diagnose chronic open-angle glaucoma by tonometry/visual fields. Screen relatives.

Treatment Immediately refer patients with acute closed-angle glaucoma to ophthalmologist for urgent IOP reduction—sight lost in hours. With chronic open-angle glaucoma, start with drugs to lower IOP—usually beta-blocker drops. Other options include pilocarpine, dipivefrin or carbonic anhydrase inhibitors. If, on follow-up, still raised IOP/visual field loss/optic nerve damage, then surgery, e.g. trabeculectomy or new laser operation.

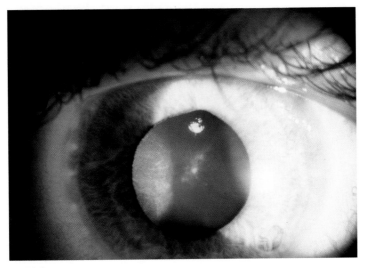

Fig. 28 A cataract.

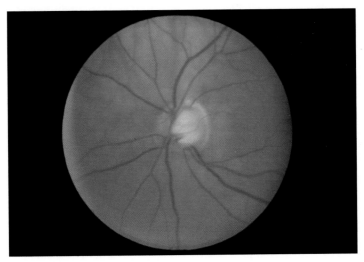

Fig. 29 The cupped optic disc in a patient with glaucoma.

Causes	Mainly viral; bacterial in <50%, e.g. *Streptococcus*, *Mycoplasma*, *Haemophilus*, and then often as secondary infection.
Diagnosis	Patient presents with cough, possibly sputum (Fig. 30A,B), and maybe febrile illness with shivering, sweating, anorexia, headache, general malaise. Dyspnoea and pleuritic chest pain may occur. Examine chest for crackles, wheezes, signs of consolidation (in pneumonia). A chest X-ray (Fig. 31) is worthwhile in patients with haemoptysis, persistent chest infections (>3 weeks, especially smokers), severe symptoms/signs, weight loss, signs suggesting other disease, immunosuppressed. Sputum culture occasionally useful, e.g. TB.
Management	(1) Antibiotics—not indicated in healthy young patients with a cough and minimal sputum. Criteria for use are: systemic illness, significant increase in sputum volume, significantly discoloured sputum, presence of chest signs or dyspnoea, persistence of chest infection (>10 days), associated heart disease or COPD, immunosuppression. Current first choice for simple chest infections is a 7-day course of amoxycillin—if penicillin allergic use erythromycin or a newer macrolide. For more serious infections, use co-amoxiclav, a cephalosporin or a new macrolide. Community-acquired pneumonia is usually *Streptococcus* but may be *Chlamydia*, *Mycoplasma* or *Legionella*—use amoxycillin plus a macrolide (for at least 2 weeks). (2) Ensure well hydrated, stop smoking, treat associated asthma/COPD. (3) Give patients with chronic cardiopulmonary disease influenza and pneumococcal vaccines.
Referral	Consider if severe symptoms/signs, other diseases, elderly, immunosuppressed, no home support. Assess patients with recurrent chest infections for cause (immunodeficiency/smoking/carcinoma/bronchiectasis etc.), unusual or resistant infections (e.g. tuberculosis), missed diagnoses (asthma/COPD/heart failure).

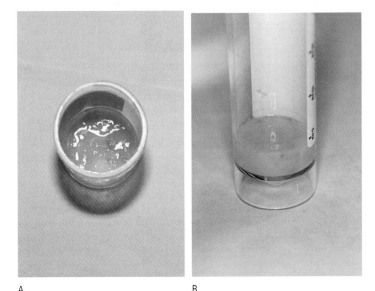

A   B

Fig. 30 (A, B) Purulent sputum indicative of a chest infection.

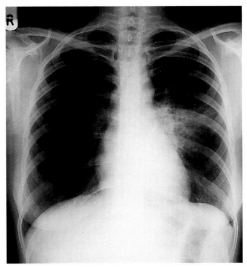

Fig. 31 Acute left-sided pneumonia on a chest X-ray.

Caused by varicella-zoster virus—lies dormant in dorsal root ganglia after chickenpox. Shingles is a reactivation of the virus.

Clinical features

Chickenpox (Figs 32 & 33).   Incubation period 21 days. Infectious 2 days before rash until last lesion crusted over. Presents with rash changing from macules to papules to vesicles and pustules. Occurs in crops, on trunk rather than peripheries. Main complication is secondary infection, but there are rare complications, e.g. pneumonia. Causes a congenital varicella syndrome.

Shingles.   Preceded by pain/tenderness, then erupts as a vesicular rash on one side of the body (Fig. 34) following path of nerve involved. May not have a rash. Complications include ophthalmic shingles and post-herpetic neuralgia (PHN). Can catch chickenpox from shingles, which is infectious until all lesions have dried over.

Treatment

Chickenpox.   Antiviral treatment shortly after onset of rash attenuates disease. Treat adults (often severely affected), children with severe attacks, the immunosuppressed, those with heart/lung disorders or significant skin disease, those with complications. Admit patients with marked respiratory symptoms, the immunosuppressed, infants, pregnant women. Pregnant women in contact with chickenpox need an antibody test and, if not immune, need varicella-zoster immunoglobulin within 4 days of exposure.

Shingles.   Antivirals within 72 h of the rash or while new lesions are forming reduce severity of attack and lessen complications; especially important for those over 50, with severe attacks, shingles of cervical, lumbar and sacral dermatomes. Refer the immunosuppressed, ophthalmic shingles, motor or sacral nerve involvement, presence of complications (neurological and severe PHN). PHN is treated with protective clingfilm/dressing, EMLA cream as local anaesthetic, TENS, analgesics, topical capsaicin, low-dose tricyclics or carbamazepine.

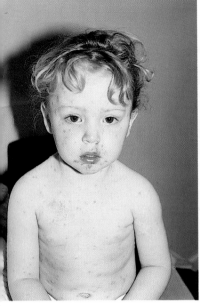

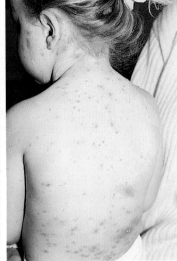

Fig. 32 Chickenpox.

Fig. 33 Chickenpox on the back.

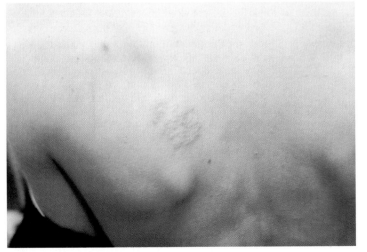

Fig. 34 The classic vesicular rash of shingles—on one side of the body following the path of a nerve.

Definition

A slowly progressive lung disease characterised by airway obstruction not changing over several months which is largely irreversible. Slight reversibility with bronchodilators but less than the >15% reversibility seen with asthma. Commonest cause is smoking.

Diagnosis

Presents with chronic progressive symptoms of cough, dyspnoea, wheeze, sputum, recurrent chest infections. May have a hyperinflated barrel chest with audible wheeze. Record airway obstruction using spirometry (Figs 35–38). In obstructive lung disease the FEV_1/FVC ratio is <70%. Key to diagnosis is measuring FEV_1 which is <80% of predicted value in COPD patients. Patients with mild COPD (symptoms mainly a 'smoker's cough') have an FEV >60% of predicted (but <80%); those with severe COPD (breathlessness a major feature) <40%. COPD is distinguished from asthma by history (smoking, age of onset, family history, atopy, trigger factors), clinical picture (chronic or exacerbations with normal intervals, sputum), evidence of airway variability/reversibility. CXR useful to exclude other pathology.

Management

Stop smoking; annual influenza vaccination; antibiotics for infections; treat associated heart failure; pulmonary rehabilitation programmes. For *mild COPD*, use beta-agonist bronchodilators or inhaled anticholinergics. For *moderate COPD*, use both and consider a trial of oral steroids (30 mg prednisolone daily for 2 weeks; if a 200 ml + ≥15% increase in FEV_1 from baseline, this is a positive response and patient will benefit from inhaled steroids). Patients with *severe COPD* benefit from all the above and may need other agents, e.g. long-acting beta-agonists, theophyllines (beware side-effects and narrow therapeutic margin), or even long-term oxygen therapy.

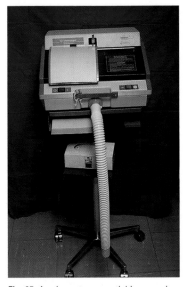

Fig. 35 A spirometer, essential in assessing patients with COPD.

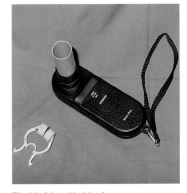

Fig. 36 A hand-held spirometer.

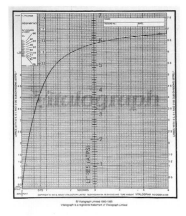

Fig. 37 A normal volume/time curve obtained using a spirometer.

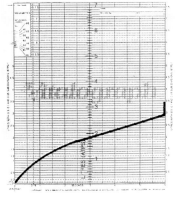

Fig. 38 A prolonged forced expiratory time—the picture of obstructive airways disease.

15 / Conjunctivitis

Causes

Inflammation of conjunctiva caused by bacteria, viruses or allergy. Rare causes: fungi, *Chlamydia.*

Diagnosis

Presents as: (1) bilateral red eyes (one eye may be affected first/more than the other); (2) irritation, itch or gritty sensation; (3) watery discharge in viral or allergic conjunctivitis, sticky yellow purulent discharge in bacterial conjunctivitis (Fig. 39: eyes often 'stuck together' in the morning). Take a history (associated allergic rhinitis, recent respiratory infection, possibility of foreign body), test visual acuity and examine conjunctiva, pupil and cornea. Distinguish from other causes of a red eye (Fig. 40). Beware unilateral red eyes, painful eyes or eyes with visual loss. In neonates purulent discharge may be caused by serious pathogens (*Chlamydia* or *Neisseria gonorrhoeae*)—swab and refer.

If patient wears contact lenses, remove and stain eye with fluorescein. If a corneal ulcer is present, refer immediately for an ophthalmological opinion; if no ulcer, treat the conjunctivitis but check contact lenses for damage and replace 10 days after infection has cleared.

Treatment

Bacterial conjunctivitis. Chloramphenicol eye drops, two drops in each eye hourly for the first day then 3-hourly, with chloramphenicol eye ointment at night, for 48 h after the eye has returned to normal. If used <7 days no real risk of bone marrow suppression. Alternative: fusidic acid drops.

Viral conjunctivitis. Aciclovir used for herpes simplex, but otherwise use chloramphenicol drops/ointment to prevent secondary infection. Refer immediately if a corneal ulcer present. *Never use steroid drops.*

Allergic conjunctivits. Use sodium cromoglycate or nedocromil drops.

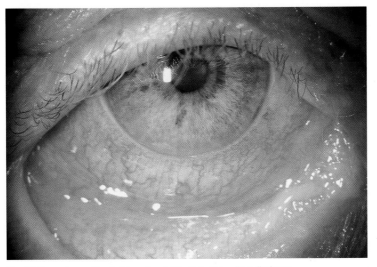

Fig. 39 The red eye of bacterial conjunctivitis. Note the yellow discharge.

	Conjunctivitis	Acute iritis	Acute glaucoma	Keratitis
Pain	Gritty	+	Severe	Variable
Vision	Normal	Blurred	Reduced	Variable
Discharge	+	Watery	None or slight	Watery + discharge
Site of redness	Peripheral	Circumcorneal	Diffuse	Diffuse or circumcorneal
Pupil size	Normal	Small	Dilated oval	Normal
Pupil response to light	Normal	Poor	Fixed	Normal
Cornea	Clear	Clear + deposits		

Fig. 40 Causes of a red eye.

Causes

Cough is the commonest reason for consulting a family doctor. Causes include: (1) upper respiratory tract infection, e.g. viral illness; (2) lower respiratory tract infection, e.g. chest infections, pneumonia; (3) lung diseases, e.g. associated with COPD, fibrosing alveolitis, cystic fibrosis; (4) smoking; (5) asthma; (6) heart failure; (7) drugs, e.g. ACE inhibitors; (8) inhaled foreign body; (9) lung cancer (Fig. 41); (10) reflux oesophagitis—may cause nocturnal cough. Remember tuberculosis (Fig. 42)!

Diagnosis

Depends on age of patient and history. In older patients consider lung disease, carcinoma (in a smoker), heart failure, late-onset asthma. In children, asthma commonly presents as a recurrent, exercise-induced or nocturnal cough. Other causes of childhood cough include infection, inhaled foreign body, anatomical anomalies, immune disorders, gastro-oesophageal reflux, cystic fibrosis, psychogenic cough. History includes type of cough, duration (>3 weeks usually significant), diurnal variation (? worse at night), relation to exercise, production of sputum, haemoptysis, associated fever/wheeze/weight loss/breathlessness/chest pain/night sweats. Take a smoking and drug history.

Examine for signs suggesting heart failure or carcinoma and then examine for local or generalised chest signs. Investigations range from reversibility testing for suspected asthma to chest X-ray for those with more serious symptoms or signs (weight loss, haemoptysis, localised consolidation, finger clubbing etc.).

Management

Depends on diagnosis. Patients with an ACE inhibitor cough can be changed to an angiotensin II antagonist. Advise re. smoking. If an antibiotic is not indicated (see chest infections, p. 23) use a cough linctus for a dry cough associated with a simple viral illness.

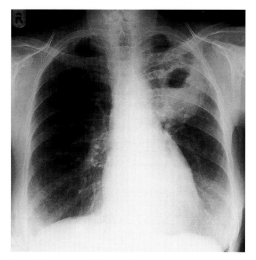

Fig. 41 Carcinoma of the lung (left upper lobe).

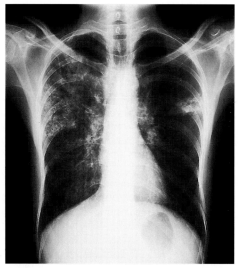

Fig. 42 Tuberculosis. Cavitation is a typical feature.

Croup (laryngotracheobronchitis), commonly caused by parainfluenza virus, causes stridor in children, typically between 6 months and 5 years.

Diagnosis

Presents with 1 or 2 days prodromal coryzal illness followed by onset of barking cough and loud inspiratory stridor—no fever, with child otherwise well. Distinguish from epiglottitis, bacterial tracheitis, inhaled foreign body. Epiglottitis usually occurs in age range 2–7, caused by *Haemophilus influenzae*, and the child looks systemically ill with rapid (hours) onset of a fever (>38°C), stridor (quieter than croup), sore throat, drooling of saliva, dysphagia and child prefers to sit upright. Bacterial tracheitis is a febrile illness with a toxic child and severe stridor.

Assessment

Severe croup can cause significant airways obstruction—symptoms necessitating immediate hospital admission are cyanosis, drowsiness, restlessness, a rising tachycardia, intercostal recession, continuous stridor or stridor at rest. Admit to hospital those under a year, where child cannot be safely monitored at home, suspected epiglottitis, bacterial tracheitis and those with an inhaled foreign body that can not be dislodged by mechanical means. *Never attempt to examine the throat of a child with stridor—this can precipitate complete airways obstruction*. In complete respiratory obstruction, tracheostomy may be needed.

Treatment of croup

Usually mild and treated by sitting child in a steamy bathroom. Nebulised adrenaline (1:1000) for emergency use in severe croup (patients still need hospitalisation). Also of use are nebulised budesonide or oral dexamethasone. Remember to review patient if using a nebuliser (Figs 43 & 44), and to instruct parents how to monitor child and recall for a further consultation if deterioration occurs.

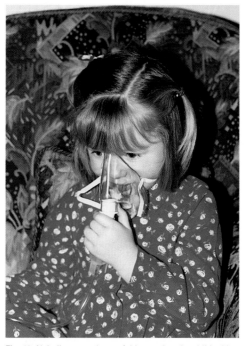

Fig. 43 Nebulisers can be useful in treating the child with croup.

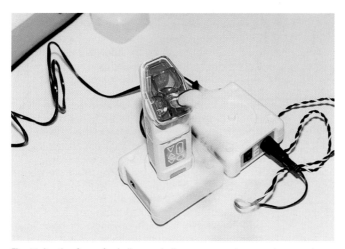

Fig. 44 Another form of nebuliser—nebulisers can come in many shapes and sizes.

'Cystitis' is used for symptoms of dysuria and frequency. Only 50% of women with cystitis have significant bacteriuria ($>10^5$ organisms/mL urine). UTI (symptoms plus bacteriuria) is commonly caused by *Escherichia coli*.

Diagnosis

Symptoms of UTI include dysuria, frequency, urgency, haematuria, nocturia, loin/suprapubic pain, smelly urine. With kidney infection, possibly rigors, fever. In children it may be non-specific, e.g. just fever. Investigate with midstream urine (MSU, Fig. 45) but not routinely necessary for adult women where UTI does not result in renal damage and is commonly precipitated by sexual intercourse; it is worthwhile for other groups, including pregnant women. Stick testing can be helpful if symptoms are present—test for protein, blood, nitrite and leucocytes (Fig. 46; absence of all four virtually excludes UTI).

Management

Encourage fluids. For uncomplicated UTI in a non-pregnant woman use a 3-day course of trimethoprim or a cephalosporin; use 7-day courses for: kidney infections, gross haematuria, pregnant women, children, males, diabetics, the immunosuppressed, underlying anomalies. Routine follow-up not required for adult women but refer the following for an opinion/investigation (IVP, Fig. 47; ultrasound, Fig. 48; cystoscopy, etc.): children, males, those who have had pyelonephritis, women with very frequent UTIs (every 2–3 months), those with gross haematuria. For recurrent cystitis ($\geqslant$4 attacks/year): document MSUs; ensure no gynaecological causes; look for precipitating factors (oestrogen deficiency, intercourse); advise (voiding/washing after intercourse, use lubricants, single-dose antibiotic post-intercourse, avoid deodorants/bath additives, wear stockings not tights/cotton not nylon underwear); try 6-month prophylactic courses of nightly 100 mg trimethoprim or 100 mg nitrofurantoin.

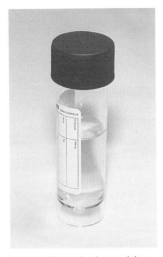

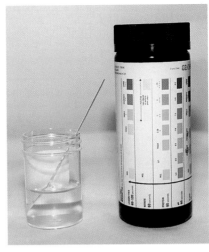

Fig. 45 MSU in a bottle containing boric acid preservative. It is important to instruct the patient how to collect the specimen.

Fig. 46 Stick testing for blood, protein, nitrite and leucocytes.

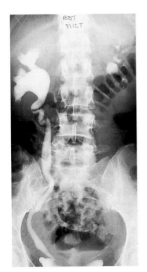

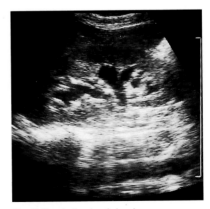

Fig. 48 Renal ultrasound showing hydronephrosis.

Fig. 47 IVP (intravenous pyelogram). Taken post-micturition, a right ureteric stone has caused obstruction at the vesicoureteric junction.

Dementia is a >6 months decline in memory, thinking and intellectual function sufficient to impair a patient's activities in daily living.

Causes

About 50–60% cases are due to Alzheimer's disease (AD), with vascular dementia and Lewy body dementia causing most of the rest. AD characterised pathologically by plaques and neurofibrillary tangles (Figs 49 & 50). Cerebral infarcts can appear on a CT Scan (Fig. 51) in vascular multi-infarct dementia.

Diagnosis

In the early stages, main features are short-term memory loss/forgetfulness. Later, memory loss worsens, patient becomes disorientated, and personality and behaviour change. Eventually affects washing, dressing, continence, ability to converse. In advanced stages, patient is restless, wandering, subject to falls with physical deterioration. AD is slowly progressive. Vascular dementia pursues a stepwise course. Use scores, e.g. Mini-Mental State Examination, Abbreviated Mental Test Score, Clifton Orientation Scale. Differentiate from depression or an acute confusional state. Exclude reversible causes of dementia (alcoholism, B_{12} deficiency, normal pressure hydrocephalus, hypothyroidism). Conduct a full (including neurological) examination, order a full blood count, ESR/plasma viscosity, blood glucose, B_{12}/folate, thyroid tests.

Management

Refer: the young (<65); those with unusual symptoms; for diagnosis if doubt; if reversible cause suspected; for management of behavioural problems; for new drugs. Management involves teamwork (GP, nurse, community psychiatric nurse, occupational therapist, physiotherapist, social worker, etc). Support carers. Treat depression (avoid tricyclics). For vascular dementia, address risk factors (diabetes, obesity, smoking, hypertension) and prescribe aspirin. Cholinesterase inhibitors can improve cognition in mild or moderate dementia due to AD.

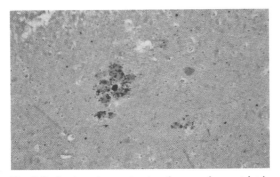

Fig. 49 Senile plaque in a postmortem tissue specimen—stained with antibody to TAU protein and red alkaline phosphatase reaction (×350).

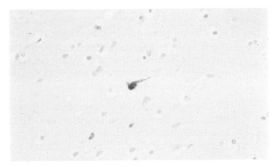

Fig. 50 A neurofibrillary tangle in a postmortem tissue specimen. Brown DAB reaction (×600).

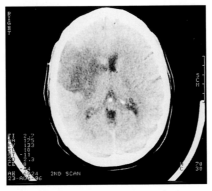

Fig. 51 CT scan showing extensive cerebral infarction in the territory of the right middle cerebral artery.

Diagnosis

Depressed patients (Fig. 52) commonly present with: feeling depressed or bursting into tears during a consultation; feelings of guilt, hopelessness, worthlessness, loss of interest, loss of libido/impotence, poor concentration; anorexia, weight loss; tiredness—'tired all the time'; sleep disturbance—classically early morning waking; hypochondriasis and multiple consultations for assumed illness; temper, aggression or retardation.

Take a history of (1) precipitating factors (relationships, work etc.); (2) past/family history depression; (3) home circumstances; (4) associated ill health, including alcohol abuse; (5) suicidal intent—have they considered self-harm/made suicidal plans? Exclude a physical cause, e.g. for weight loss. Remember depression in the elderly (affects 15% of the over-65s).

Management

(1) Explain—nature of depression; it is treatable but drugs may take up to 3 weeks to work. (2) Listen and support, involving family, friends, counsellor, community psychiatric nurse. Consider cognitive therapy, psychotherapy. (3) Prescribe drug treatment for moderate to severe depression, if biological features (e.g. weight loss, early waking), psychotic symptoms, recurrent/persistent depression. Refer to psychiatrist if suicidal intent, bipolar depression, severe postnatal depression, failure to respond to treatment. (4) Use adequate antidepressant doses, continue course for 6 months then withdraw over 2–3 months—if three trials of antidepressant fail, consider long-term treatment. (5) Follow-up patient regularly, monitoring compliance. Warn re. side-effects. (6) Selective serotonin reuptake inhibitors and selective noradrenaline reuptake inhibitors are preferable to tricyclics—they are as effective, safer in overdose, do not potentiate alcohol and have fewer side-effects.

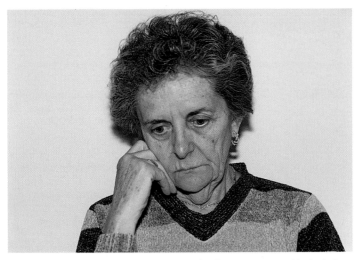

Fig. 52 A patient with depression. The depressed patient may present with physical symptoms like tiredness as well as feeling depressed.

21 / Diabetes mellitus

Definition

Disorder characterised by hyperglycaemia resulting from relative/absolute insulin lack; >80% have non-insulin dependent diabetes mellitus (NIDDM).

Diagnosis

IDDM presents with history (days or weeks) of thirst, polyuria, nocturia, weight loss. Can present with ketoacidosis—dehydration, drowsiness, deep sighing respirations, ketones on breath/in urine. NIDDM usually in older patient, more gradual onset with (1) non-specific problems, e.g. tiredness, recurrent infection, pruritus vulvae; (2) asymptomatic glycosuria; (3) diabetic complications (feet (Fig. 53), vascular disease, retinopathy (Fig. 54), neuropathy, nephropathy). Confirmed by repeated fasting plasma glucose level >7 mmol/L. Patients with fasting plasma glucose level 6.1–6.9 mol/L have impaired fasting glucose.

Management

(1) Patient education. (2) Prevent complications (assess feet, blood pressure, lipids, renal function, fundi, neuropathy). (3) Monitor random blood glucose (should be <10 mmol/L), glycosylated haemoglobin (should be in normal range). (4) Diet important—aim for >50% of calories from carbohydrate (<35% from fat).

Insulin. Required as emergency for ketoacidosis. Most young patients need insulin and many NIDDM patients eventually require insulin. Human insulin is standard. Traditional = twice daily regime of short- and intermediate-acting: now many use multiple injection regimes. Counsel re. injection technique (Fig. 55), hypos, use of glucagon, never to stop insulin. Fat hypertrophy (Fig. 56) at sites causes erratic absorption—rotate sites.

Drugs for NIDDM. If a trial of diet (2–3 months, unless very hyperglycaemic) is unsuccessful, add oral drugs. Sulphonylureas usually first line but can cause weight gain, hypoglycaemia. Metformin used for obese with no renal impairment, liver or cardiac disease. Acarbose used for postprandial hyperglycaemia.

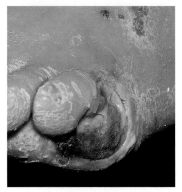

Fig. 53 Critical ischaemia in a diabetic foot.

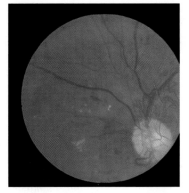

Fig. 54 A proliferative diabetic retinopathy.

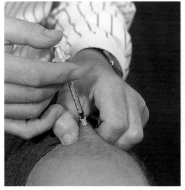

Fig. 55 Injecting insulin into the thigh.

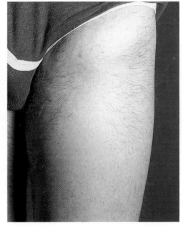

Fig. 56 Lipohypertrophy.

An increased frequency and fluidity of the stools. Causes of acute diarrhoea: infection (commonest), anxiety, alcohol, drugs, diverticulitis, colitis. Chronic diarrhoea (>2 weeks) can be infective but exclude bowel pathology.

Diagnosis

In *acute diarrhoea*, rests on history (duration, foreign travel, bloody diarrhoea, contacts with diarrhoea, recent drugs, vomiting, pyrexia, abdo pain, frequency of motions, recent dietary indiscretion, food handler). Abdominal examination rarely helpful but assess degree of hydration and request a stool sample (Fig. 57) if (1) food handler; (2) recent foreign travel; (3) bloody diarrhoea; (4) diarrhoea >10 days; (5) patient systemically ill; (6) immunosuppressed; (7) severe symptoms; (8) works in an institution; (9) suspected food poisoning. In *chronic diarrhoea*, focus on rectal bleeding, abdominal pain, weight loss and symptoms suggesting malabsorption, with full examination (including rectal) and investigation/referral depending on suspected pathology.

Management

In adults with acute diarrhoea, maintain hydration with 'copious fluids' and oral rehydration solutions (Fig. 58). Solids reintroduced as appetite allows. For mild socially inconvenient diarrhoea, use loperamide. Antibiotics indicated for travellers' diarrhoea (acute/prophylaxis), severe *Salmonella*, *Shigella*, *E. coli* or *Campylobacter* infection, *Clostridium difficile*, giardiasis. Children with acute diarrhoea managed with oral rehydration solutions—avoid antidiarrhoeals. In infants with diarrhoea and/or vomiting, look for signs of dehydration (loss of skin elasticity, weight loss, oliguria, sunken eyes, sunken fontanelle, dry mouth, irritability). If signs of dehydration admit; otherwise advise no milk for 24–48h, using an oral rehydration solution instead. Review within 24h (earlier if condition deteriorates). If improving, begin to regrade through quarter to half to three-quarter to full-strength feeds in 12–24h steps.

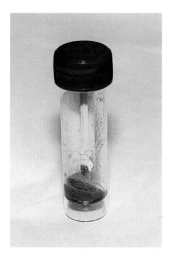

Fig. 57 A stool sample.

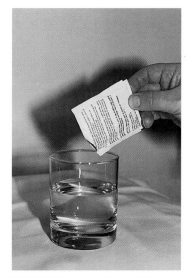

Fig. 58 Making up an oral rehydration solution. Use of rehydration solutions is a key part of the management.

Diverticula (Figs 59 & 60) are outpouchings of mucosa and serosa through the muscular wall of the colon and are present in a third of patients under 60 and over half by the age of 70.

Diagnosis

Most diverticula are asymptomatic but diverticular disease can present with: (1) diverticulitis (inflammation of diverticula) with pain, fever and abdominal tenderness—complications include perforation with peritonitis, abscess and fistulae formation; (2) rectal bleeding—can be massive; (3) intestinal obstruction; (4) colicky abdominal pain, usually situated in the left iliac fossa and relieved by defaecation, associated with a change in bowel habit. These are the commonest symptoms. To confirm the diagnosis and exclude other pathologies, notably bowel cancer (Fig. 61), requires a sigmoidoscopy and barium enema (possibly a colonoscopy if there is a high index of suspicion of a neoplasm).

Management

(1) Patient with complications may need hospital admission. (2) Surgery, often emergency surgery, may be required for abscesses, fistulae, obstruction, perforation, peritonitis, stricture, significant haemorrhage. (3) Medical management of diverticular disease includes: antispasmodic drugs to relieve the pain of the abdominal colic; lactulose occasionally needed for constipation; a high-fibre diet, possibly with the addition of artificial sources of fibre.

Diverticular disease is rare in those eating a high-fibre diet, the fibre acting by lowering the intraluminal pressure. While a high-fibre diet will not cause existing diverticula to disappear, it will prevent further progression of the disease and may help alleviate the symptoms of abdominal colic and constipation.

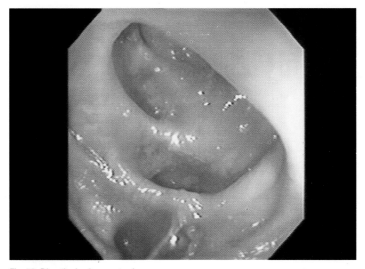

Fig. 59 Diverticula shown at colonoscopy.

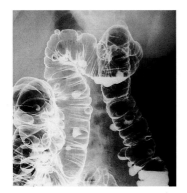

Fig. 60 Diverticula on a barium enema.

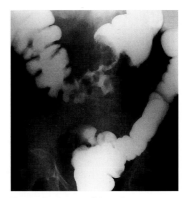

Fig. 61 Carcinoma of the colon on a barium enema—note the obstruction to the flow of barium in the middle of the slide.

Diagnosis

Presents with epigastric pain relieved by food and antacids, often waking patient at night and radiating to back. DU runs a relapsing course with weeks of pain interspersed with asymptomatic periods. Gastric ulcers and gastric cancer are less common—suggested by symptoms of weight loss, anorexia, vomiting. DU complications include perforation and haemorrhage (Fig. 62). Epigastric tenderness may be present on examination. Exclude bleeding (ask about stool colour and include rectal examination for melaena if suspected). Endoscopy (Fig. 63) confirms diagnosis and allows biopsy for *Helicobacter pylori* (HP) (Figs 64 & 65). HP can also be tested by serology. For a single attack of dyspepsia in a patient under 45 with no serious symptoms (bleeding, vomiting, anaemia, weight loss, dysphagia, abdominal mass, severe pain), try a short trial of treatment, resorting to endoscopy if not resolving. If patient HP-positive, sensible to try eradication therapy; if HP-negative reassure patient that a DU is unlikely. All patients over 45 with new onset dyspepsia and those under 45 with serious symptoms merit endoscopy.

Management

(1) Stop smoking. (2) Avoid NSAIDs, aspirin. (3) Reduce alcohol intake. (4) Treat, eradicating HP. Over 95% of DUs are HP-positive; eradicating HP reduces recurrence and complications. Eradicate HP with 1 week triple therapy (a proton pump inhibitor (PPI) and two antibiotics); this achieves at least 90% eradication. To heal an acute DU, prescribe 4 weeks PPI, with 1 week being in the form of triple therapy. If symptoms recur after treatment, test to ensure HP eradication via a breath test. Gastric ulcers require endoscopic confirmation of healing; DUs do not. (5) Acute complications may require surgery.

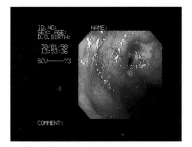

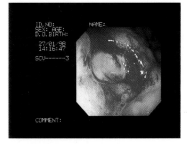

Fig. 62 A duodenal ulcer at endoscopy with a clot over the site (this DU bled).

Fig. 63 A non-bleeding duodenal ulcer at endoscopy.

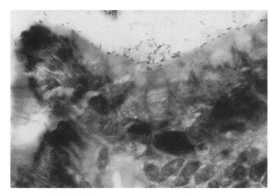

Fig. 64 *Helicobacter pylori* bacteria on the gastric mucosa (slide stained with modified Giesma).

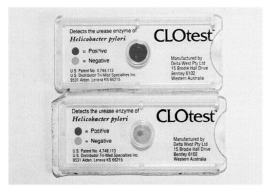

Fig. 65 CLO test. A gastric mucosal biopsy, taken at endoscopy, is tested for *Helicobacter*—positive, red; negative, yellow.

Dysmenorrhoea

Primary dysmenorrhoea—painful periods, usually in young women, with no underlying pelvic pathology—is treated by reassurance, analgesia, oral contraception or NSAIDs. Secondary dysmenorrhoea is associated with endometriosis, pelvic inflammatory disease and fibroids (Fig. 66).

Menorrhagia

Causes and diagnosis

Menorrhagia is excessive menstrual loss (>80 mL per period). Causes include fibroids, endometriosis, polyps, endometrial carcinoma, blood disorders, hypothyroidism, IUDs (Fig. 67), dysfunctional uterine bleeding (due to no local pathology). Take a history to confirm menorrhagia—clues are the need for double sanitary protection (towels and tampons), using a towel on the bed at night, using nappies, clots and flooding. Ask re. intermenstrual or postcoital bleeding; perform a pelvic examination and smear (if indicated); take a full blood count. Serum iron and thyroid function tests may be required. Women under 40 with menorrhagia do not need referring to exclude carcinoma (very rare < age 40). Occasionally acute-onset menorrhagia in a younger patient is due to a polyp, necessitating referral. Over 40 referral is required for hysteroscopy and biopsy and possibly ultrasound to exclude other pathology. Outpatient endometrial sampling (Fig. 68) is now often used, to both monitor and manage patients with menorrhagia.

Treatment

Depends on diagnosis. The most effective drugs are the combined oral contraceptive, NSAIDs, antifibrinolytics (e.g. tranexamic acid) and danazol (a second choice if the other three fail). In future, the levonorgestrel intrauterine system (Fig. 69) may be licensed for menorrhagia. Progestogens are not as effective. Surgical options include endometrial resection or ablation using laser or hysterectomy.

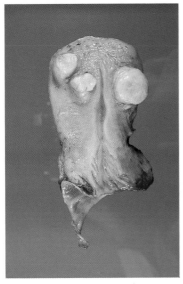

Fig. 66 A uterus with three fibroids clearly shown.

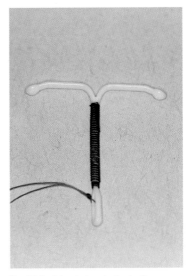

Fig. 67 An intrauterine device (coil).

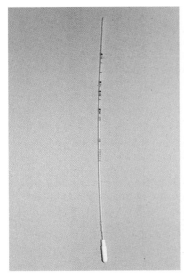

Fig. 68 A Pipelle de Cornier tube used for taking an endometrial biopsy.

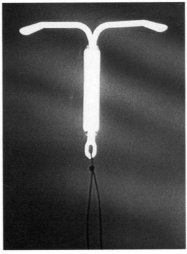

Fig. 69 The levonorgestrel intrauterine system.

Ear wax

Wax (Fig. 70), a common cause of impaired hearing, is diagnosed on auriscopic examination. Prior to syringing, advise patients to use olive oil drops twice a day for 3 days. Do not syringe if drum is perforated. Pull the pinna of the ear upwards and backwards and direct a flow of water (body temperature) upwards and backwards along the canal—do not aim at the drum!

Otitis externa (Fig. 71)

Presents with itching (main symptom), discharge and impaired hearing. Usually bilateral. Predisposing causes: trauma, foreign body, eczema/psoriasis, diabetes, swimming, certain occupations.

Management

(1) Consider predisposing causes (remember foreign body if unilateral in a child!). (2) If minimal debris and you can see an intact drum, treat with 2 weeks antibiotic/steroid drops or spray. (3) If debris present, remove from ear canal, e.g. with a wax hook or Jobson Horne probe, before prescribing antibiotic/steroid drops (if drum intact). If you can't see the drum or there is a perforation present, refer. Advise patient to avoid swimming for several weeks.

Referral

- With gross debris you may need referral for suction under the microscope.
- If resistant to the above treatment, may need referral. Consider: (1) overgrowth by fungi as in Figure 72 (take swab and treat with antifungal drops); (2) a missed cause, e.g. diabetes; (3) a missed middle ear disease with perforation and discharge (usually there is more discharge than with otitis externa and the discharge is unilateral); (4) hypersensitivity to the antibiotic/steroid drops.
- If there is surrounding cellulitis, refer urgently for i.v. antibiotics.

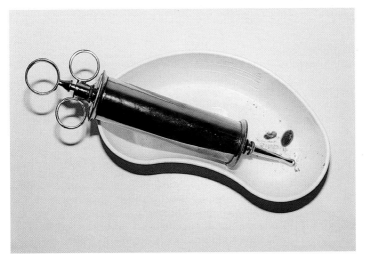

Fig. 70 Ear wax and an ear syringe.

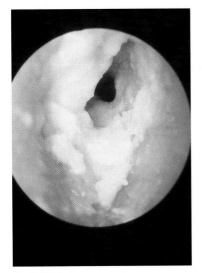

Fig. 71 Otitis externa.

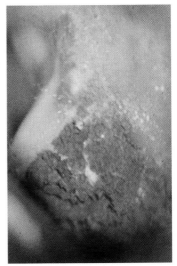

Fig. 72 A fungal otitis externa.

Diagnosis

Eczema (Figs 73–75) is an inflammatory skin condition presenting as a red, itchy, scaly rash. In the acute stage, blisters and vesicles occur. The commonest form is atopic eczema, genetically determined and linked with asthma/allergic rhinitis, usually starting in infancy (face affected) or childhood (affecting elbows, knees, neck, wrist, ankles). Other forms are seborrhoeic eczema (infants—cradle cap/nappy rash; adults—scalp, face, trunk), discoid eczema, venous (stasis) eczema, pompholyx (blisters on hands and feet), asteatotic eczema (a dry eczema in the elderly) and exogenous or contact eczema resulting from contact with an irritant/allergen (often work-related).

Management

Atopic eczema. (1) Reassure and explain. Wear cotton not wool. Consider house dust mite avoidance measures. (2) Avoid soap and detergents. (3) Use emollients regularly and frequently as creams/ointments, soap substitute and bath oil. (4) Treat infection with antibiotics (or an urgent antiviral if eczema herpeticum). (5) Use sedative antihistamines at night short-term if severe pruritus. (6) Use topical corticosteroids (not if virally infected)—ointments for dry scaly eczema, creams for weeping lesions. Use the least potent giving control, e.g. 1% hydrocortisone for children. May need moderately potent or potent steroids for short-term treatment of acute exacerbations. Never use more than 1% hydrocortisone on face. (7) If not resolving on these strategies, refer for hospital treatment (azathioprine, cyclosporin, UVB phototherapy, oral steroids).

Seborrhoeic eczema. Yeast infection important and topical antifungals combined with hydrocortisone are useful. Try ketoconazole shampoo for the adult scalp. In infants use emollients, 1% hydrocortisone and antifungals.

Contact eczema. Need to identify cause—patch testing useful.

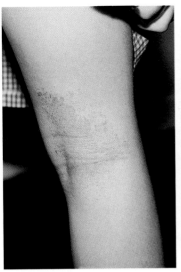

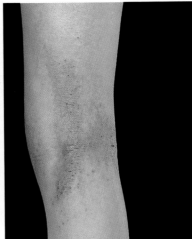

A   B

Fig. 73 (A, B) Atopic eczema in the popliteal fossa—a common site.

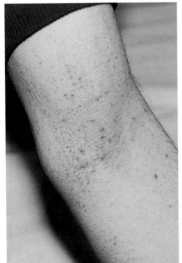

Fig. 74 Atopic eczema in the antecubital fossa—another common site.

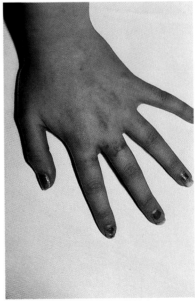

Fig. 75 Allergic contact dermatitis where rings have been worn.

Epilepsy is a tendency to recurrent seizures. Types: (1) generalised seizures including (a) tonic-clonic seizures (possible aura, then unconsciousness followed by tonic muscle spasm, jerking, possible tongue biting/urinary incontinence and postictal headache/drowsiness/confusion) and (b) absences (in children, last seconds—stare vacantly before resuming activity); (2) partial seizures, e.g. temporal lobe epilepsy, where disturbance of consciousness results in variety of symptoms. Febrile convulsions occur in 3% of children (usually aged 6 months–6 years, tonic-clonic seizures, lasting <5 min).

Diagnosis

Largely on history—best from eyewitness. Distinguish a seizure from a faint. Examination usually normal. Epilepsy idiopathic in 70% of patients but exclude a cause (e.g. head injury, meningitis, encephalitis, alcohol, drugs, cerebrovascular disease, tumours). Refer to neurologist for further tests—EEG (see Figs 76 & 77), scans etc.

Management

A single seizure does not constitute epilepsy. *Acute management*: protect airway; if convulsion prolonged, use diazepam. For *childhood febrile convulsion*, ensure clear airway, use paracetamol and tepid sponging to lower temperature, rectal diazepam (Fig. 78) to stop convulsion, seek the cause. Refer if in doubt and if first febrile convulsion. *Chronic epilepsy management* involves (1) reviewing diagnosis; (2) patient education/advice re. driving, lifestyle, contraception; (3) drug therapy to control recurrent seizures—75% can be controlled on one drug. Ensure right drug for seizure type, correct dose regimen, patient compliance (monitoring side-effects may need blood tests and anticonvulsant levels, particularly with phenytoin). After a 3-year seizure-free period, consider phased withdrawal of treatment. Prophylactic anticonvulsants for children with febrile convulsions no longer recommended.

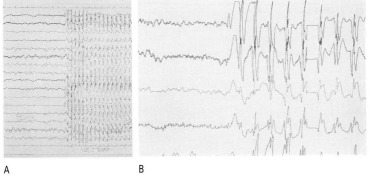

A   B

Fig. 76 (A) Petit mal epileptic seizure manifesting as an absence attack. This EEG tracing shows the characteristic 3 cycle/s spike and wave activity. (B) Close-up of (A).

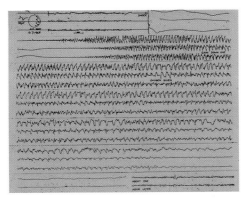

Fig. 77 EEG tracing of a focal-onset epileptic seizure becoming secondarily generalised.

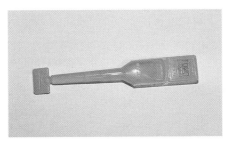

Fig. 78 A diazepam rectal unit dose applicator for acute treatment of convulsions. The top is removed before use.

Causes | Children usually bleed from Little's area (Fig. 79) on anterior part of the septum: infection, nose-picking, foreign body are common causes.
In adults, common causes are polyps, trauma, posterior bleeds in older patients (check for hypertension). Rare causes: tumours, bleeding tendency.

Assessment | A severe bleed, often in the elderly, can cause major blood loss and require a transfusion. Assess blood loss, ask re. infection, unilateral or bilateral bleeds, past medical history and any drugs prescribed. In the elderly measure the blood pressure; in children look for a foreign body.

Management | *Acute epistaxis.* Advise patient to sit with the head bent forwards, and to compress the soft part of the nostrils together continuously for 15 min, breathing through the mouth. An ice pack applied to the bridge of the nose may help. If after 15 min the bleeding continues, nasal packing or a balloon is necessary. A Merocel expansile nasal pack (Fig. 80) is useful; once inserted, it expands to form a tampon within the nose when in contact with blood. If packing fails to control bleeding, arterial ligation may be required.

Recurrent epistaxis. Exclude a cause. In a younger patient (bleeding from the Little's area), use chemical cautery (refer the under-4s). First anaethetise the area with a pledget of cotton wool soaked in local anaesthetic or a lignocaine nasal spray, then apply a silver nitrate stick (Fig. 81) for about 10 seconds until the septum blanches. Never cauterise both sides of the septum (danger of perforation). Warn the patient they may get a nose bleed within 24 h of cautery. If chemical cautery fails, refer to hospital.

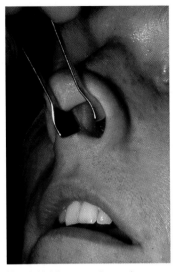

Fig. 79 Little's area on the nasal septum.

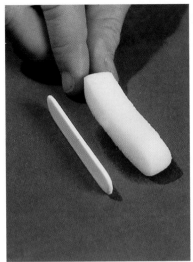

Fig. 80 Merocel expansile nasal packs (pre- and post-expansion).

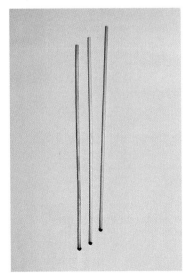

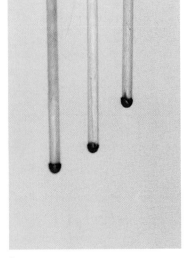

A

B

Fig. 81 (A) Silver nitrate sticks for nasal cautery. (B) Close-up of the tips.

Causes (Fig. 82)

Commonest cause is psychological (depression, anxiety); <10% of patients have an underlying physical cause. Most common physical cause is anaemia. Remember also drugs (e.g. beta-blockers), viral infections (e.g. glandular fever), postviral fatigue, hypothyroidism and diabetes. Malignancies constitute <1% of patients presenting with tiredness.

Diagnosis

The history should first concentrate on the psychological, seeking a positive diagnosis of anxiety and/or depression. If there are no confirmatory psychological symptoms, ask about any recent viral illness, sore throat, cough, polyuria/polydipsia, breathlessness, palpitations, weight loss. Explore any physical symptoms volunteered by the patient. Take a drug history. Beware the patient with weight loss—depression and malignancy can cause tiredness and are often associated. Patients with no anxiety/depression merit an initial screen of full blood count (Fig. 83), plasma viscosity/erythrocyte sedimentation rate, urine test for sugar and protein and consideration of thyroid function tests and a test for glandular fever. The patients should be seen within 2 weeks for results, when further physical examination/tests/referral can be considered.

Chronic fatigue syndrome. Also termed myalgic encephalomyelitis, this has a prevalence as high as 1%. The pattern is of 6 months or longer fatigue interfering with the patient's daily functioning, with associated symptoms such as impaired concentration/memory, sleep disturbance, myalgia, arthralgia, headaches, sore throat and lymphadenopathy. The fatigue may initially have arisen after an acute infection. There is no diagnostic test. Over 80% recover spontaneously. Treatment options include graded exercise programmes and cognitive behaviour therapy.

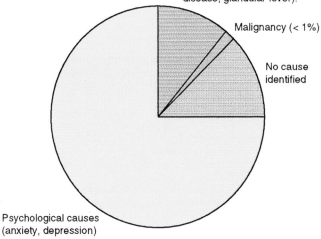

Physical causes (anaemia, drugs, hypothyroidism, diabetes, post viral fatigue, cardiovascular, renal, hepatic disease, glandular fever).

Malignancy (< 1%)

No cause identified

Psychological causes (anxiety, depression)

Fig. 82 Causes of fatigue.

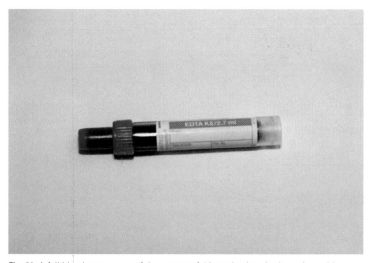

Fig. 83 A full blood count—one of the most useful investigations in the patient with fatigue when no diagnosis of anxiety/depression can be made.

31 / Gastro-oesophageal reflux disease (GORD)

GORD is used to describe symptoms and/or mucosal damage resulting from reflux of gastric contents into the oesophagus.

Diagnosis

History of: (1) retrosternal burning sensation (heartburn), worse after food or lying flat; (2) regurgitation of acid gastric contents into mouth; (3) less commonly odynophagia (pain on swallowing), belching, cough (from aspirated gastric contents), hoarseness. Symptoms suggesting serious pathology/complications (e.g. stricture, carcinoma; Figs 84 & 85) include weight loss, dysphagia, vomiting, anaemia and haematemesis; these patients require endoscopy. Symptoms of GORD do not correlate well with endoscopic findings (Fig. 86)—about half of GORD patients have a normal endoscopy (these need oesophageal pH monitoring). Initially treat on the basis of a history, including relief from antacid. Endoscope those with the significant symptoms noted above and first-onset dyspepsia in the patient over 45.

Management

(1) Lifestyle—lose weight; stop smoking; avoid large meals/food before bedtime/spicy or fatty foods; reduce alcohol/tea/coffee intake; avoid stooping/bending; do not wear tight clothes; raise head of bed. (2) Antacids and alginates used for mild GORD do not heal the oesophagitis. (3) H_2 receptor antagonists are more effective, but the most effective drugs for acid suppression are the proton pump inhibitors (PPIs) which can heal 80% of patients with oesophagitis in 4 weeks, and 90% in 8 weeks. (4) Prokinetic agents like cisapride are also used.

Over 75% of GORD patients relapse within 6 months of stopping treatment and most require either further courses of therapy or long-term maintenance treatment, usually with a PPI. Patients with complications of GORD—stricture or Barrett's oesophagus—require long-term PPI therapy. Young patients with severe GORD may need anti-reflux surgery.

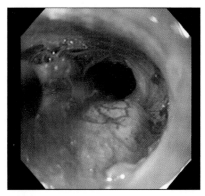

Fig. 84 A balloon dilator passing through a benign oesophageal stricture at endoscopy.

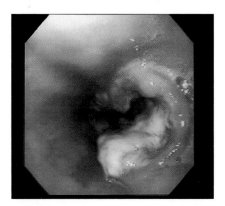

Fig. 85 An ulcerating carcinoma of the lower oesophagus seen at endoscopy.

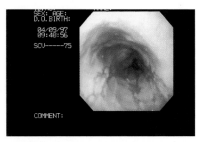

Fig. 86 Oesophagitis at endoscopy.

Haemorrhoids (piles)

A haemorrhoid (Fig. 87) is an enlarged pad of venous blood-filled tissue. Causes include straining at stool, constipation, pregnancy. Patients present with bleeding (exclude carcinoma), prolapse, itching, fullness after defaecation, pain, discomfort. Observe externally or with a proctoscope. Perform a rectal examination, but haemorrhoids may not be palpable. Treat minor non-prolapsing haemorrhoids with a high-fibre diet (plus bulking agents as required) together with a topical steroid/local anaesthetic ointment or suppositories if discomfort or itching. For larger, bleeding or prolapsing internal (above the dentate line) haemorrhoids, treatment includes infrared coagulation, injection with oily phenol, rubber band ligation or haemorrhoidectomy.

Pruritus ani

Causes include poor hygiene, haemorrhoids, prolapse, fungal infection, threadworms, skin diseases, anorectal discharge, fissure or fistula (Fig. 88). Carry out a full (including rectal) examination to determine cause. Advise careful washing after defaecation followed by gentle drying, avoiding scratching, short-term use of topical steroid/local anaesthetic ointments. Treat any cause.

Rectal bleeding

Causes usually local anorectal conditions, e.g. haemorrhoids, fissures, pruritis ani, prolapse. Exclude carcinoma/polyps. Take a history (is blood just on toilet paper or darker mixed with stool; is there a change in bowel habit?). Examine patient, including external examination, rectal examination and proctoscopy. Further investigation required, including sigmoidoscopy (Figs 89 & 90), if no cause found or the history suggests serious pathology.

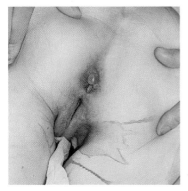

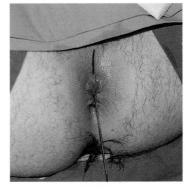

Fig. 87 Posterior external haemorrhoid (and anterior anal skin tag).

Fig. 88 Anal fistula.

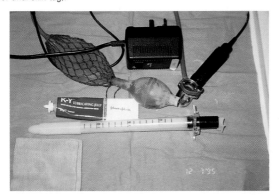

Fig. 89 Sigmoidoscopy tray showing sigmoidoscope and lubricating jelly.

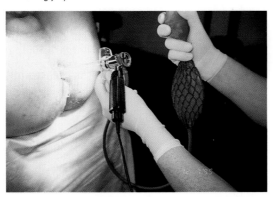

Fig. 90 Sigmoidoscopy being carried out.

Definition and prevalence

Hay fever is a seasonal allergy to pollen/mould spores. Allergic rhinitis (prevalence 15%) consists of seasonal allergic rhinitis and perennial allergic rhinitis (PAR). Symptoms of allergic rhinitis are nasal blockage, rhinorrhoea and sneezing. Allergic rhinitis is associated with other atopic conditions, e.g. eczema, asthma.

Clinical features

Hay fever. Allergic rhinitis (itchy, runny nose, sneezing), conjunctivitis (red, itchy, watering eyes), pollen asthma (wheezy chest) in May–July for grass pollen—earlier or later with other pollens/spores.

Perennial allergic rhinitis. All-year-round symptoms—often get secondary sinusitis, postnasal drip, loss of sense of smell. Examine the nose for signs of a rhinitis (Fig. 91) and to exclude other pathology, e.g. polyps (Fig. 92). A blood RAST (radioallergosorbent) or skin prick test can identify allergens, commonly house dust mite (Fig. 93).

Management

Avoid the allergen. Treatment options: (1) Newer, non-sedating, once daily oral antihistamines. Beware drug interactions. Not used in pregnant women. Relieve sneezing/rhinorrhoea but not nasal blockage. (2) For allergic conjunctivitis use sodium cromoglycate eye drops. (3) For allergic rhinitis (including PAR) once daily topical nasal corticosteroids are most effective. Demonstrate use. With hay fever start treatment before season begins. A trial for allergic rhinitis should be 6–8 weeks. Long-term use is safe with standard doses. (4) For severe hay fever disrupting exams/life events, a course of oral steroids is justified. Depot steroid injections inflexible and can cause muscle wasting. (5) Treat associated asthma. (6) Desensitisation procedures risk fatal anaphylaxis—only use in hospital with resuscitation facilities available.

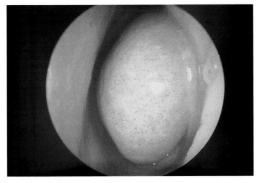

Fig. 91 Allergic rhinitis: hypertrophied inferior turbinate with secretions.

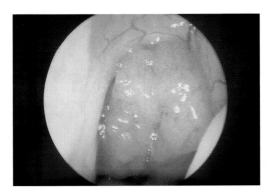

Fig. 92 Nasal polyps filling the nasal cavity.

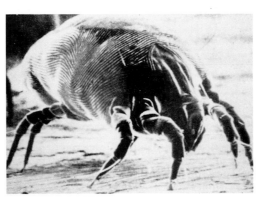

Fig. 93 The house dust mite.

Headache

Causes

Commonest causes are viral illness/sinusitis, tension headache, migraine. Remember sudden-onset headache of meningitis, cerebral haemorrhage, glaucoma, severe hypertensive encephalopathy and the less acute headache of temporal arteritis, brain tumour.

Diagnosis

Rests on history—character, severity, site of pain, sudden onset or chronic, associated symptoms, associated anxiety/depression, previous attacks, triggers. A brain tumour is rare (progressive morning headache/vomiting).

Migraine

Differentiate from tension headache (bitemporal, 'pressure'/'band', lasts days/weeks, no associated symptoms), but can have both. Migraine is an episodic 'pulsating' headache, usually unilateral (Fig. 94), lasting 4–72 h and associated in 70% of cases with nausea/vomiting (may also be photophobia). Examination is normal. 70% have family history. Up to 20% patients have an aura preceding headache which may be visual (double vision, zigzag lines etc.) or sensory/motor/speech disturbance. The triggers are listed in Fig. 95.

Treatment of migraine

Reassure; identify triggers.

Acute attack.   First try simple analgesics (paracetamol/aspirin) early in the attack, possibly with anti-emetic; NSAIDs also worth a trial. If simple analgesia is ineffective or migraines severe, use (if no contraindications or drug interactions) a 5HT agonist—this rapidly relieves both headache and vomiting (warn patient re. side-effects).

Prophylaxis.   If attacks severe (or >3 months) consider beta-blockers (e.g. propranolol), pizotifen or low-dose amitriptyline. Need at least a 3-month trial of prophylactic—try withdrawal after 6–12 months.

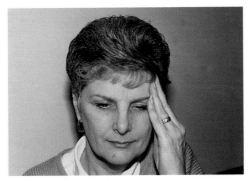

Fig. 94 The patient with migraine typically has a unilateral pulsating headache, lasting 4–72 h and associated with nausea.

FOOD	Chocolate, cheese, citrus fruits, red wine, coffee
LIFESTYLE	Dieting, missed/irregular meals, over exertion, travel shiftwork, lack of sleep, oversleeping, smoking
PSYCHOLOGICAL	Stress, worry, anger, anxiety, depression, excitement
ENVIRONMENT	Television, excess heat/noise/light
HORMONAL	Menses (menstrual migraine), menopause, HRT, combined oral contraceptive

Fig. 95 Common trigger factors of migraine.

35 / Heart failure

Results from reduced cardiac output insufficient to meet body needs. Main causes: coronary artery disease and hypertension.

Clinical features

Symptoms: dyspnoea worse on exertion or lying down (orthopnoea), paroxysmal nocturnal dyspnoea, ankle swelling (Fig. 96), tiredness. Signs: raised jugular venous pressure, lung crepitations, ankle oedema, resting tachycardia, third heart sound, displaced apex beat, ascites, hepatomegaly. Investigations: full blood count, urea, creatinine, electrolytes, thyroid function, glucose, lipids, ECG, CXR (Fig. 97), echocardiogram (most useful—shows ventricle function, valve problems; Fig. 98). B-type natriuretic peptides are raised in heart failure; if low, suggests another cause.

Management

(1) Advise—no smoking; no excess alcohol; no added dietary salt; graded exercise; lose weight; avoid NSAIDs/tricyclics. (2) Establish cause, e.g. ischaemia, hypertension, valve disorder. (3) Treat risk factors, e.g. hypertension. (4) Treatment options: (a) *Loop diuretics*—monitor electrolytes; thiazides used in the mildest cases, but less potent. (b) *ACE inhibitors*—improve prognosis and symptoms. Use with non-potassium-sparing diuretics starting with low dose and working upwards. Indicated for patients with left ventricle systolic dysfunction. Check for contraindications. Refer for hospital initiation if need >80 mg frusemide daily, creatinine >150μmol/L, systolic BP < 90 mmHg, potassium >5.5 mmol/L, low serum sodium (<130 mmol/L), hypovolaemia, peripheral vascular disease. Check urea, creatinine, electrolytes before and 2 weeks after starting ACE inhibitor, stopping if significant rise in creatinine (>25% or up to 200 μmol/L) or potassium >5.5 mmol/L. Monitor renal function at 3 months then 6-monthly if stable. (c) *Digoxin*, particularly if associated atrial fibrillation. (d) *In specific patients*: anticoagulation, anti-arrhythmic drugs, low-dose beta-blockers (under consultant supervision), hydralazine and nitrates, surgery.

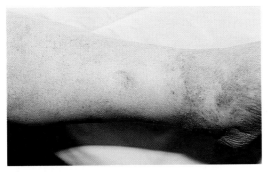

Fig. 96 Pitting ankle oedema in a patient with heart failure. Ankle swelling may be a sign of heart failure.

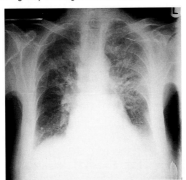

Fig. 97 Chest X-ray of a patient with heart failure showing the changes of pulmonary oedema.

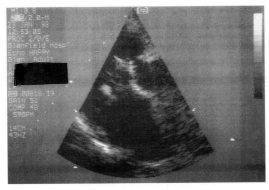

Fig. 98 An echocardiogram (showing mitral stenosis). Echocardiography is essential for the proper diagnosis and management of heart failure.

Prevalence

Ideal serum total cholesterol is <5.2 mmol/L (LDL cholesterol < 3.4 mmol/L). A raised total serum cholesterol is >6.5 mmol/L (LDL cholesterol >5.0 mmol/L). Raised triglycerides >2.3 mmol/L. HDL cholesterol protects.

Diagnosis

Signs of hyperlipidaemia: a corneal arcus (Fig. 99) at a young age, xanthelasmata and xanthomata (Figs 100 & 101). Screen, with random cholesterol, patients with existing or family history of CHD/hyperlipidaemia, diabetics, hypertensives, chronic smokers. If random cholesterol is elevated, repeat fasting, together with triglycerides, HDL and LDL cholesterol. Need at least two estimations to confirm hyperlipidaemia. Exclude secondary causes of hyperlipidaemia (hypothyroidism, renal failure, liver failure, diabetes, obesity, alcoholism, drugs which raise cholesterol, e.g. thiazides).

Management

Advise on CHD risk factors. Encourage exercise. First try 3 months of a cholesterol-lowering diet with <30% of total calories from fat—but diet only reduces cholesterol by 10–15%. If diet fails, consider drugs.
- Postmyocardial infarction—reduce LDL cholesterol to <3.2 mmol/L
- CHD present—reduce LDL cholesterol to <3.4 mmol/L
- Chol >7.8 mmol/L, no CHD risk factors—reduce LDL cholesterol to <3.4 mmol/L (check for familial hyperlipidaemia, consider referral)
- Chol = 6.5–7.8 mmol/L, no major CHD risk factors—reduce LDL cholesterol to 4 mmol/L
- Chol = 6.5–7.8 mmol/L with major risk factor for CHD (including HDL cholesterol < 0.9 mmol/L, diabetes, hypertension, poor family history)—reduce LDL cholesterol to <3.4 mmol/L
- Chol = 5.2–6.4 mmol/L—rarely need drug treatment unless major CHD risk factors.

Drugs of choice for hypercholesterolaemia are statins.

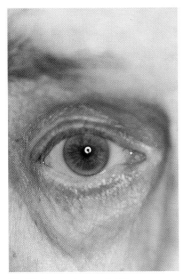

Fig. 99 A corneal arcus (in this casa a senile corneal arcus not associated with hyperlipidaemia).

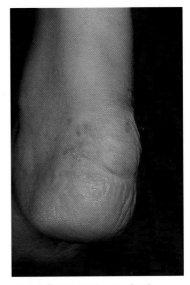

Fig. 100 Tendon xanthoma—site: the Achilles tendon.

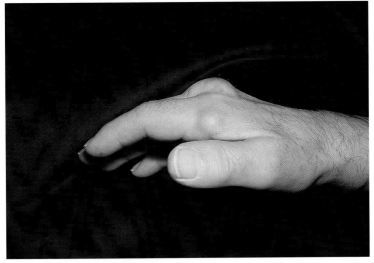

Fig. 101 Tendon xanthoma—site: the hand.

Definition

- Diastolic BP, 90–99 mmHg—borderline to mild hypertension
- Diastolic BP, 100–109 mmHg—moderate hypertension
- Diastolic BP, 110 mmHg and over—severe hypertension.
  Systolic BP, >160 mmHg is elevated. Target BP is <160/90 mmHg.

Diagnosis

Record BP accurately (Fig. 102) on at least three occasions before diagnosing hypertension: over 3–6 months if diastolic < 100 mmHg; over 4–6 weeks if 100–110 mmHg; and over 2 weeks if 110–130 mmHg. Refer urgently if over 130 mmHg. Average of three or more readings is the patient's BP. If borderline/suspected white coat hypertension consider ambulatory blood pressure monitoring (Fig. 103). All hypertensives (average BP >160/95) need an assessment of CHD risk factors, an examination (pulse, heart size, heart sounds, fundi), urinalysis, urea, electrolytes and creatinine, lipids, blood glucose, ECG. Consider a CXR.

Management

Advise—lose weight if obese; reduce salt intake; reduce excess alcohol intake; take regular exercise; stop smoking. Drug treatment for all those with diastolic >100 mmHg or sustained systolic >160 mmHg. If diastolic BP is 90–99 mmHg, treat if target organ damage (stroke, angina, cardiomegaly, retinopathy, renal failure), if major risk factors (diabetes, hyperlipidaemia, males, poor family history, smokers) or if over age 60. Tailor drug treatment to the patient. Drugs include thiazides, beta-blockers, ACE inhibitors (useful if heart failure, diabetes, LVH. Dry cough in about 15%. Monitor renal function. The angiotensin II antagonists are as effective without the cough), calcium antagonists, alpha-blockers and moxonidine.

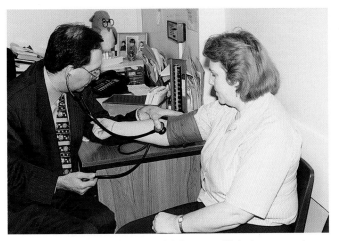

Fig. 102 Recording the blood pressure. It is important this is done accurately.

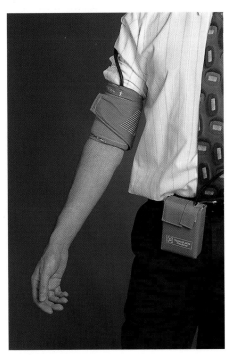

Fig. 103 A patient wearing ambulatory blood pressure monitoring equipment.

Hypothyroidism is a consequence of thyroid hormone deficiency. Major causes are listed in Fig. 104.

Diagnosis

Patients usually become hypothyroid gradually, the slow changes in symptoms/signs making diagnosis difficult. Symptoms/signs include: puffy face with periorbital oedema, lethargy, weight gain, dry skin, hair loss, impaired mental functioning (including dementia), depression, constipation, hoarse voice, menorrhagia, cold intolerance. On examination, pulse rate may be slow and reflexes may have a delayed relaxation time. May be an associated carpal tunnel syndrome and anaemia. Diagnosis is confirmed by finding the raised serum thyroid-stimulating hormone (TSH) of primary hypothyroidism, but very rarely you may find the low thyroxine/low TSH combination indicative of hypothyroidism secondary to hypothalamic-pituitary disease (these patients need referral for further investigation). Primary hypothyroidism may be associated with hypercholesterolaemia or other autoimmune diseases, e.g. pernicious anaemia. Rarely, hypothyroid patients can present with a life-threatening coma. The newborn are screened for hypothyroidism in the UK by means of blood taken by heel prick on about day 7.

Treatment

In the usual case of primary hypothyroidism, treatment is with thyroxine replacement therapy, aiming to keep the TSH in the normal range. Start young adult patients with 100 μg daily (usual adult dose, 100–150 μg) but in the older patient start with 25–50 μg, increasing slowly every 2–4 weeks towards 100 μg. In patients with heart disease start with 25 μg—thyroxine therapy can precipitate angina and arrhythmias. Measure the TSH 3 months after starting thyroxine replacement therapy, then at 6 months. Once patient is stabilised on thyroxine, an annual TSH is sufficient.

Common causes	Thyroid disease (e.g. autoimmune)
	Thyroidectomy (Fig. 105) or following radioiodine therapy
Rare causes	Congenital
	Drugs (e.g. lithium, amiodarone)
	Iodine deficiency
	Secondary hypothyroidism resulting from hypothalamic—pituitary disease

Fig. 104 Causes of hypothyroidism.

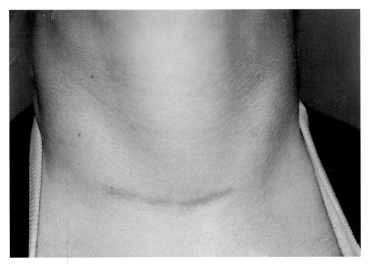

Fig. 105 A thyroidectomy scar.

Prevalence	About 10–15% of the population; more common in women.
Causes	Causes not precisely known although a disturbance of gut motility, an increased gut sensitivity to external stimuli and psychological factors may all have a role.
Definition	The 'Rome symptom criteria' now used to make a positive diagnosis of IBS (Fig. 106).
Diagnosis	Based on a history satisfying the symptom criteria listed in Fig. 106. Key features include abdominal pain relieved by defaecation, bloating and alteration of bowel habit. Examination of the patient (including rectal examination) should be normal, as should a full blood count and an erythrocyte sedimentation rate/plasma viscosity. Sigmoidoscopy is regarded by many as essential, but with typical symptoms in a younger patient most family doctors will try treatment first. Symptoms outside these criteria, e.g. weight loss, rectal bleeding, nocturnal diarrhoea, positive findings on examination or symptoms in a patient over 40, will merit referral for further blood tests, sigmoidoscopy and consideration of a barium enema/colonoscopy. Patients with IBS have no specific structural abnormalities diagnosed on sigmoidoscopy or colonoscopy (Fig. 107).
Treatment	Reassure the patient, then treat symptomatically: for *constipation* try a high-fibre diet (Fig. 108)/bulk forming agents; for *diarrhoea* try a high-fibre diet, loperamide; for *abdominal colic* try antispasmodics, peppermint oil or tricyclics; for *bloating* try a low-fibre diet, peppermint oil.
	Treat any underlying anxiety/depression. Psychological therapies (including hypnotherapy) may help. Dietary modification is also of value (look for dietary precipitants of symptoms, e.g. caffeine, milk products, wheat, alcohol).

- At least 3 months continuous or recurrent symptoms of abdominal pain relieved by defaecation and/or associated change in stool frequency or consistency

And two or more of the following on at least a quarter of occasions or days.

- Altered stool frequency
- Altered stool form (lumpy/hard or water/loose)
- Altered stool passage (straining/urgency/feeling of incomplete emptying)
- Passage of PR mucus
- Bloating or a feeling of abdominal distension

Ref. Thompson WG, Creed F, Drossman DA, Heaton JW, Mazzacca G 1992 Functional bowel disorders and functional abdominal pain. Gastroenterol Int 5: 15–91

Fig. 106 Symptom criteria of irritable bowel syndrome.

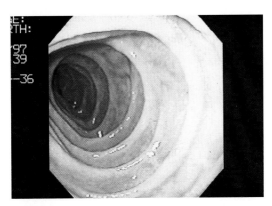

Fig. 107 Normal colon observed at colonoscopy.

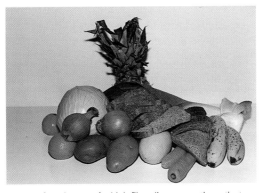

Fig. 108 Constituents of a high-fibre diet: ensure the patient has written information material.

Acute injury

A history (mechanism of injury, site of pain, swelling, locking, clicking, giving way) and examination (swelling or effusion, site of tenderness, passive/active movements) should help diagnosis. A swelling within hours of injury is a haemarthrosis (refer); 80% have an *anterior cruciate ligament (ACL) injury*. Tests for cruciate ligament injury are the draw test (Fig. 109) and Lachman's test (Fig. 110). ACL damage may cause a painless giving way of the knee. History of twisting while weight-bearing suggests a *torn meniscus*—the effusion usually appears the next day and can get locking (i.e. the patient cannot fully extend the knee—refer), tenderness in the joint line (Fig. 111), clicking on movement and a painful giving way of the knee. McMurray's test may confirm (Fig. 112—may get a painful click with a meniscus tear). *Collateral ligament injuries* are common, the patient presenting with an effusion and tenderness over the site of the ligament—test for laxity by valgus then varus stressing of the knee.

Minor knee injuries are managed with ice packs, NSAIDs and a Tubigrip bandage—review in 7 days. For major meniscus/cruciate ligament tears, investigations include MRI scan and arthroscopy.

Non-traumatic knee pain

Causes include anterior knee pain syndrome, osteoarthritis, pseudogout, gout, rheumatoid arthritis, septic arthritis. Chondromalacia patellae presents as pain over the patella with tenderness on pressing the patella's articular surface. Osgood–Schlatter's disease presents in children with pain, tenderness and swelling at the tibial tuberosity. If the knee is normal on examination, remember that pain from the hip and lower spine can be referred to the knee.

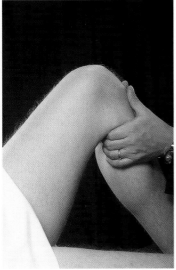

Fig. 109 Anterior draw test: with hamstrings relaxed and foot steadied, pull the tibia forwards.

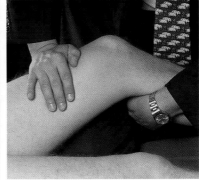

Fig. 110 Lachman's test: knee rested over examiner's thigh, distal femur steadied and tibia lifted upwards.

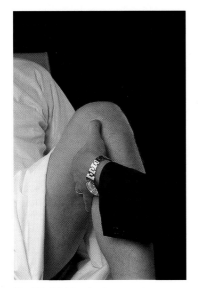

Fig. 111 Joint line tenderness.

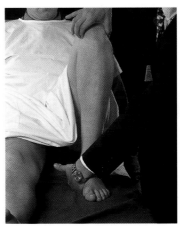

Fig. 112 McMurray's test: patient's knee flexed and finger and thumb on the joint line, rotating the tibia on the femur.

Common lumps include:
- *Ganglion*—a smooth, jelly-like lump usually on the dorsum of the wrist or foot. If large enough to produce symptoms, it can be removed.
- *Lipoma*—a benign fatty tumour which can occur anywhere in the body; again, can be surgically removed if large enough to produce symptoms.
- *Sebaceous cyst* (Figs 113 & 114)—the cyst contains a fatty secretion and is topped by a punctum. Common on the back and scalp. Surgical removal is the treatment.

Ingrowing toenails (Fig. 115) are painful, often with infection of the surrounding tissue. Treatment is by a wedge resection, although recurrent ingrowing toenails may need a total nail ablation, removing the germinal matrix.

Moles

Moles are very common but it is important to distinguish a benign mole/seborrhoeic keratosis (Fig. 116) from a malignant melanoma. Symptoms/signs suggesting a malignant melanoma are: recent change in the size of a skin lesion; irregular shape of the skin lesion; change in pigmentation, with variation/irregularity of the colour; inflammation, crusting or oozing of the lesion; bleeding of the lesion; itching.

In men, the back is the commonest site for a malignant melanoma; in women it is the lower leg. Refer any pigmented lesions with the above characteristics for excision/histology. The prognosis of malignant melanoma depends on the tumour thickness when diagnosed and it is curable in the early stages. Educate your patients re. 'mole-watching'. Benign naevi can be excised, but again send all lesions for histology.

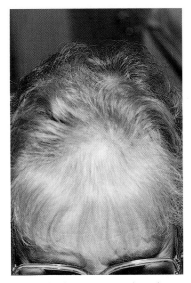

Fig. 113 A sebaceous cyst on the scalp from above.

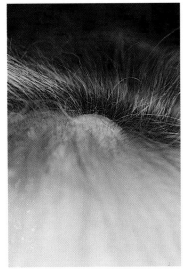

Fig. 114 A sebaceous cyst on the scalp from the side.

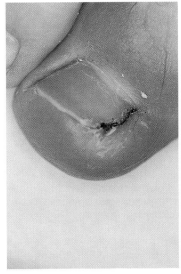

Fig. 115 An ingrowing toenail.

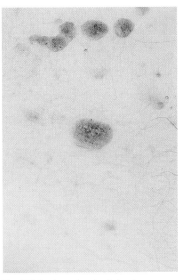

Fig. 116 Benign seborrhoeic keratoses.

Tinea

Fungal skin infection affecting: (1) body (*tinea corporis*)—ringed lesions ('ringworm') with a red raised scaly edge spreading outwards and a clear centre; (2) groin (*tinea cruris*)—similar lesion spreading outwards on upper thigh; (3) foot (*tinea pedis, athlete's foot*, Fig. 117)—usually a macerated, itchy, interdigital scaling of 4th/5th toes, spreading onto surface of foot; (4) nail (*tinea unguium*, Fig. 118)—usually the toenails which look thickened, discoloured (yellowish/brownish) and separated from the nail bed (onycholysis); (5) scalp (*tinea capitis*)—usually in children, presents with an inflamed, pustular lesion (kerion) or as a scaling alopecia.

Diagnosis

Typical rash. To confirm examine skin scrapings/ nail clippings microscopically and can culture.

Treatment

Advise—do not share towels; open not tight-fitting footwear. Some forms, e.g. corporis, capitis, caught from animals. For small localised patches use a topical imidazole or terbinafine cream. For larger patches and nail or scalp infections, use oral therapy with terbinafine (2–6 weeks for tinea pedis, 4 weeks for tinea corporis, 6 weeks–3 months for fingernails, 3–6 months for toenails) or itraconazole therapy; neither recommended for children.

Nappy (diaper) rashes

Napkin (diaper) dermatitis (Fig. 119). Erythema due to wet soiled napkins appearing on buttocks, inner upper thighs, genitalia and lower abdomen, sparing skin creases. Treatment: barrier creams, frequent changing of disposable nappies (diapers).
Candidiasis. Red patches with scaling edges, pustules, satellite lesions and involving flexures. Treatment: topical imidazole.
Seborrhoeic eczema. Diffuse red rash involving flexures, associated with seborrhoeic eczema elsewhere. Treatment: 1% hydrocortisone cream preferably combined with an antifungal.

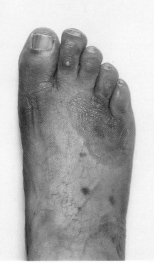

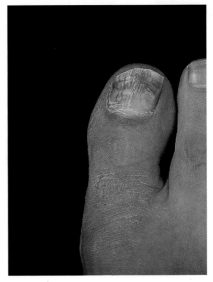

Fig. 117 Tinea pedis (tinea of the foot). **Fig. 118** Tinea unguium tinea of the nail.

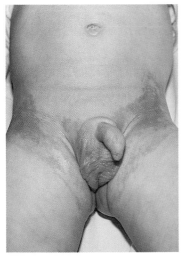

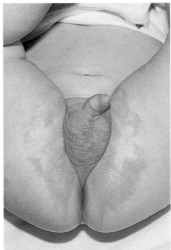

A

B

Fig. 119 (A, B) Napkin (diaper) dermatitis.

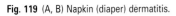

Definition

Calculate the patient's body mass index (BMI) [weight (kg)/height^2 (m^2) (Fig. 120)]. A patient of height 1.83 m and weight 74 kg would have a BMI of 74/1.83^2 = 22. A BMI of 20–24.9 is normal; 25–29.9 is overweight; $\geqslant$30 is obese. The girth–height ratio (waist circumference divided by height) estimates central obesity—associated more with heart disease risk than BMI.

Risks

Increases morbidity and mortality from heart disease since obesity is associated with hypertension, hyperlipidaemia, non-insulin-dependent diabetes and lack of exercise. Associated with osteoarthritis, gout, menstrual problems, gall bladder disease and certain cancers.

Diagnosis

Based on the above measurements, but remember to exclude hypothyroidism Cushing's disease (rare) and drugs causing weight gain (tricyclics, danazol, etc.).

Management

(1) Diet—reduce calorie intake; standard diets are 1000–1200 kcal/day for women, 1500 kcal/day for men. Change the diet by increasing fibre content, reducing fat and sugar intake and eating complex carbohydrates. (2) Behaviour modification—behavioural therapy, changing eating patterns, useful. (3) Exercise programmes. (4) Drugs—Appetite suppressants have so far suffered from an unacceptable risk of side-effects but new drugs being developed. (5) Surgery—consider for the severely obese (BMI > 40). (6) Group therapy—in the doctor's surgery or with commercial organisations. Weight loss is easy in the first weeks of any programme. The key to successful management lies in maintaining weight loss, which requires regular follow-up by the nurse/therapist/group.

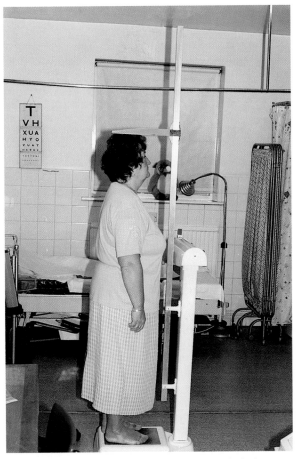

Fig. 120 Measuring the height and weight to determine the body mass index.

Characterised by loss/erosion of cartilage and associated bone changes, including hypertrophy, cyst and osteophyte formation. Risk factors: age, family history, past trauma and obesity (for OA knee).

Clinical presentation

Initially joint pain (worse on movement, relieved by rest) and stiffness. With time, limitation of movement, tenderness and crepitus on movement and, finally, joint deformity and instability. Sites commonly affected are hands (giving rise to Heberden's and Bouchard's nodes, Fig. 121), hips, knees (Fig. 122), cervical and lumbar spine.

Diagnosis

Based on history, examination (limited movement, joint tenderness, crepitus, bony swelling, deformity), negative blood tests (normal C-reactive protein/erythrocyte sedimentation rate/plasma viscosity, negative rheumatoid factor) and typical X-ray findings (joint space narrowing, osteophytes, subchondral cysts/sclerosis; Fig. 123). X-ray findings may not correlate with clinical symptoms.

Management

(1) Explain nature of osteoarthitis and its course. (2) Advise—lose weight; specific exercises to improve muscle strength around joints. (3) Physiotherapy—exercise programmes, ultrasound, heat, hydrotherapy, etc. (4) Use of aids, e.g. aids to walking, special shoes. (5) Occupational therapy to install aids in patient's home. (6) Drugs—try simple paracetamol type analgesia (with or without codeine) first. For associated joint inflammation, try NSAIDs particularly if joint swelling present. NSAIDs can cause GI bleeding, renal impairment and exacerbation of asthma. New NSAIDs inhibiting the COX-2 enzyme produce less GI/renal side-effects. NSAID use should be monitored, the patient using them intermittently rather than on long-term repeat prescription. Intra-articular steroid therapy can produce significant improvement if inflammation/effusion present. (7) Surgery—hip and knee replacement surgery (Fig. 124) useful for patients with severe pain or instability.

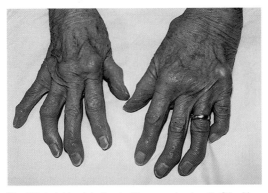

Fig. 121 Arthritis of the hands. Shows predominantly OA with some features of rheumatoid arthritis at the MCP joints.

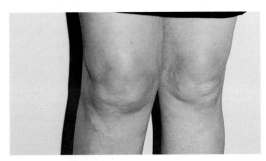

Fig. 122 Osteoarthritis of the right knee.

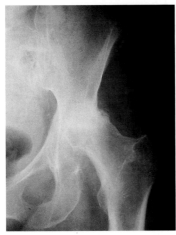

Fig. 123 Osteoarthritis of the hip on X-ray.

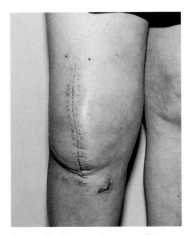

Fig. 124 Total knee replacement of the knee in Fig. 122.

Definition | A disease characterised by low bone mass resulting in low trauma fractures. Women more at risk. Bone mass decreases with age.

Risk factors | Risk factors for developing osteoporosis include: a previous low trauma fracture, a family history of osteoporosis, an early menopause (natural or surgically induced), premenopausal amenorrhoea > 6 months, prolonged immobilization; use of long-term steroids (>7.5 mg daily over 6 months), thyrotoxicosis; hyperparathyroidism; malabsorption, vitamin D/calcium deficiency, rheumatoid arthritis, chronic liver disease, alcoholism, smoking, lack of exercise, low body mass index, hypogonadism in men.

Diagnosis | Osteoporosis is a 'silent' disease, being usually asymptomatic until a fracture occurs. Common osteoporotic fracture sites: the hip, vertebrae and wrist. Symptoms/signs following a fracture include: back pain, kyphosis (Fig. 125) or loss of height. Changes on a plain X-ray occur late in the disease. The best method for assessing bone loss (and fracture risk) is by bone densitometry (Figs 126 & 127), most commonly by means of dual X-ray absorptiometry (DXA). Osteoporosis can be diagnosed if the bone density is at least 2.5 standard deviations below the mean reference value for a normal premenopausal woman. Once osteoporosis diagnosed look for secondary causes/risk factors.

Management | (1) Advice—exercise; good dietary intake of calcium and vitamin D; avoid excess alochol intake and smoking. (2) HRT is the main preventative and can slow bone loss if osteoporosis present. (3) Calcium and vitamin D supplements benefit those who are deficient, e.g. the housebound elderly. (4) Biphosphonates inhibit bone resorption; particularly useful for older women not wishing HRT. (5) Calcitonin by injection or intranasal route (not yet in UK) also used.

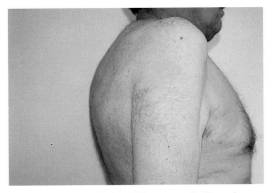

Fig. 125 Kyphosis in a patient with osteoporosis. The patient had a wedge fracture of the vertebra.

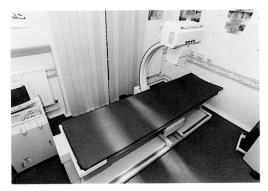

Fig. 126 An imaging densitometer.

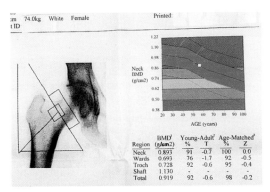

Region	BMD[1] (g/cm2)	Young-Adult[2] %	T	Age-Matched[3] %	Z
Neck	0.893	91	-0.7	100	0.0
Wards	0.693	76	-1.7	92	-0.5
Troch	0.728	92	-0.6	95	-0.4
Shaft	1.130	-	-	-	-
Total	0.919	92	-0.6	98	-0.2

:m 74.0kg White Female   Printed:
t ID

Neck BMD (g/cm2)

AGE (years)

Fig. 127 A bone densitometry report.

Acute otitis media (AOM)

AOM (Fig. 128) is a middle ear infection, usually in children under 10 and following an upper respiratory tract infection.

Diagnosis

Child usually presents with earache with or without pyrexia. Hearing reduced. On examination initially an injection of vessels of the handle of the malleus, proceeding to a red drum which bulges and finally perforates (with ear discharge).

Treatment

Analgesia. Paracetamol.
Antibiotics. Evidence that early antibiotics reduce duration/severity of symptoms or prevent complications is poor. Decide a policy, e.g. use antibiotics for those children: (1) under age 3 (higher risk of complications); (2) with persistent discharge post-perforation; (3) with recurrent attacks (consider low-dose prophylaxis or intermittent treatment); (4) systemically ill with pyrexia; (5) with symptoms persisting > 3 days; (6) where it is difficult to arrange a follow-up. Treat with a 3-day course of broad-spectrum antibiotic. Follow up children with discharge, recurrent attacks or suspected hearing loss 4 weeks after an attack. If the drum or hearing is still abnormal at 3 months, refer for audiometry etc.

Otitis media with effusion (glue ear) (Fig. 129)

Child presents with a conductive hearing loss or disturbed school behaviour. Earache usually mild, if present, Many detected via screening. Drum is dull grey/yellow with no light reflex and possibly a fluid level behind.

Treatment

May spontaneously resolve. Try 8 weeks' antibiotics. The Otovent device is useful in children over 5. If persisting after about 3 months, refer for grommet (Fig. 130) insertion (possibly with adenoidectomy). Grommets usually stay in 6–12 months before being extruded and improve hearing.

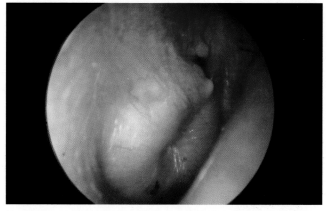

Fig. 128 Acute otitis media. (From Drake-Lee 1995: *Clinical otorhinolaryngology*, Churchill Livingstone, with permission.)

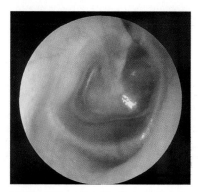

Fig. 129 Otitis media with effusion (glue ear).

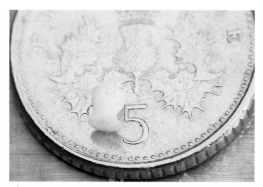

Fig. 130 A grommet on a 5 pence piece.

Clinical features

A chronic condition associated with: *bradykinesia*—slow movements, expressionless face, stooped posture (Fig. 131); *tremor*—initially unilateral, 'pill rolling', present at rest, improved by movement; *rigidity*—'cogwheel' rigidity; *gait disturbance*—shuffling gait, loss of arm swing, festination; *other features*—dribbling of saliva, increased sweating, constipation, micrographia, monotonous speech, depression, impaired postural reflexes, recurrent falls.

Tendon and plantar reflexes normal. Diagnosis is clinical (exclude drug-induced Parkinsonism) and assisted by a positive response to levodopa.

Management

Explanation and practical help in daily living from nurse, physiotherapist, occupational therapist, social worker, speech therapist.

Drug treatment. Options include: (1) Levodopa with a dopa decarboxylase inhibitor is a mainstay of treatment (build up dose gradually over weeks) but has two problems: (a) after about 5 years the effects begin to wear off and the patient may experience an 'on/off' effect, fluctuating between mobility and immobility; (ii) side-effects (nausea/vomiting, postural hypotension, involuntary movements, psychiatric symptoms). (2) Anticholinergics help tremor but not bradykinesia. Side-effects limit use. (3) Selegiline has a dopaminergic action, can be combined with levodopa therapy but there is debate over its use. (4) Dopamine agonists generally less effective than levodopa. Many different preparations—tend to be used (a) as monotherapy or adjuncts to low-dose levodopa in younger patients (to try and delay levodopa use); (b) as an adjunct to levodopa therapy to counter the 'on/off' effect. (5) COMT inhibitors (block the breakdown of levodopa) can be used to improve symptoms in patients on long-term levodopa. (6) Apomorphine—inject subcutaneously.

Surgery. Stereotactic surgery is a final option.

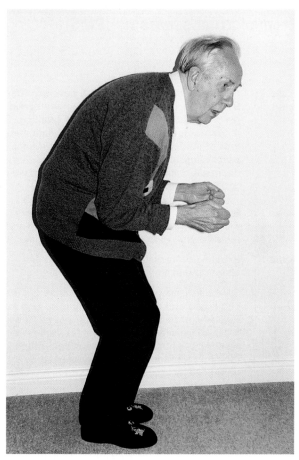

Fig. 131 The stooped posture of Parkinson's disease.

Prevalence and diagnosis

About 5–10% of all women are severely affected. Symptoms include: fluid retention with weight gain, a bloated feeling and breast swelling/tenderness; headaches, lethargy, constipation, loss of libido, clumsiness, sleep disturbance; psychological problems—irritability, tension, depression, anxiety, poor concentration, violent or aggressive behaviour.

A symptom diary is useful for diagnosis. Symptoms should be worse in the 2 weeks before a period and relieved by menstruation. No blood tests helpful. Exclude a depressive illness.

Management

Explain and reassure. General measures: encourage exercise and a healthy diet.

Specific drug treatment. Options include: (1) The combined oral contraceptive pill (Fig. 132) may help (if contraception required), but not always and it can make symptoms worse. (2) Depression may respond well to a selective serotonin reuptake inhibitor. (3) Mastalgia can be relieved by gamolenic acid in evening primrose oil (Efamast) or bromocriptine. (4) Use of oestradiol implants or oestrogen patches (Fig. 133) together with progesterone. (5) Progestogens, e.g. norethisterone 5 mg twice daily from day 19 to 26 or dydrogesterone 10 mg twice daily from day 12 to 26, may be tried but may not give a consistent improvement. Some gynaecologists use the progestogen only pill.

Refer. For those with more severe symptoms, or where the above treatment fails, refer to a gynaecologist for a consideration of: (1) danazol (but side-effects include fluid retention); (2) a gonadotrophin-releasing hormone analogue—cures symptoms of PMS but replaces them with menopausal ones requiring oestrogen; (3) surgical oophorectomy followed by oestrogen replacement therapy.

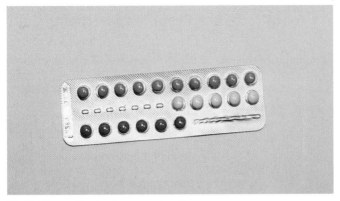

Fig. 132 The combined oral contraceptive pill.

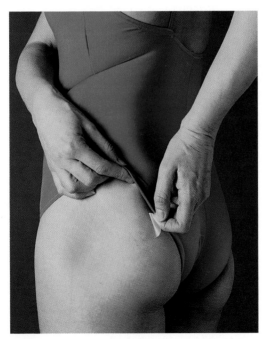

Fig. 133 An oestrogen patch. Although oestrogen patches are used by gynaecologists, the patch shown is not licensed as such for treating premenstrual syndrome.

49 / Prostatic hyperplasia (hypertrophy)

Diagnosis

Benign prostatic hyperplasia (BPH, Figs 134 & 135) affects a third of men over 50. Diagnosis is made from symptoms, either obstructive (poor stream, hesitancy, terminal dribbling, incomplete bladder emptying) or irritative (frequency, urgency, nocturia). International Prostate Symptoms Score grades symptom severity based on seven symptoms—feeling of incomplete bladder emptying, frequency of micturition (urinating <2-hourly), straining to start micturition, stopping and starting, urgency (difficulty postponing micturition), poor stream, nocturia. With a significant score, perform a rectal examination (if normal, does not exclude BPH but may detect a hard, irregular carcinoma), test urine, take an MSU, renal function tests and blood for prostate specific antigen (PSA) in the under-75s. A PSA in the normal range (0.5–4 ng/mL) is reassuring, whereas most of those with a PSA > 10 ng/mL will have prostate cancer.

Management

Refer to specialist.   Refer those with severe symptoms, urinary retention, a palpable bladder, suspected prostate carcinoma, haematuria, urinary tract infections, renal impairment. Patients with mild symptoms and no complications may prefer to await events.

Medical treatment.   An option for those with uncomplicated mild to moderate BPH. Prescribe: (1) alpha-blockers, which relax smooth muscle, acting rapidly to relieve symptoms but do not shrink prostate; or (2) finasteride, which can reduce prostate size (best for large prostates), reducing complications of urinary retention and need for surgery.

Surgery (usually transurethral resection prostate, Fig. 136). Required for those with severe obstructive symptoms, haematuria, urinary retention, recurrent urinary tract infection, renal impairment secondary to BPH, bladder stones, no response to medical therapy.

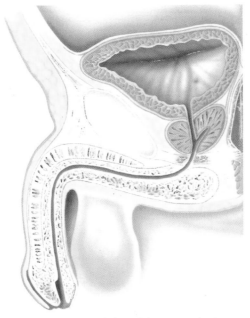

Fig. 134 Anatomy and relations of the prostate gland.

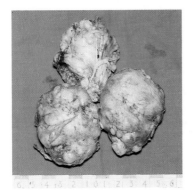

Fig. 135 A surgically removed enlarged prostate.

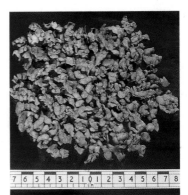

Fig. 136 Chippings from a surgically resected prostate.

Prevalence

Affects 2% of population. There is a familial factor and it can be precipitated by trauma, drugs, infection, stress.

Clinical presentation

Commonest form is *plaque psoriasis*—well-defined pink/red plaques with silvery scales (Fig. 137) usually found on elbows (Fig. 138), knees (Fig. 139), scalp. May only affect scalp and may involve nails (with pitting, onycholysis) and joints (causing an arthropathy). Less common forms include: (1) *guttate psoriasis*—a widespread eruption of small plaques, often following infection; (2) *pustular psoriasis*; (3) *flexural psoriasis* of axillae, groins, submammary area and natal cleft; (4) *erythrodermic psoriasis*—a serious generalised erythema affecting whole body and requiring emergency admission.

Management

Explanation—treatable, not infectious, does not scar. Four main treatments: (1) Vitamin D analogues—first-line treatment for the plaques of mild to moderate psoriasis. Scalp preparations also available. (2) Short contact therapy with dithranol preparations—used for stable plaques, but some patients very sensitive to dithranol. (3) Tar-based preparations—old preparations messy but, alone or combined with salicylic acid, often used for scalp psoriasis. Recent doubts about possible carcinogenic potential. (4) Topical steroids—use limited by side-effects (cutaneous atrophy, adrenal suppression, infection) and may get a severe rebound exacerbation when stopped. Valuable for treating psoriasis in the flexures, genitalia, scalp, hands and feet, face (mild topical steroids only).

Emollients may also be used to help control the scaling and reduce the irritation of mild psoriasis.

Referral

For those with severe psoriasis or psoriasis resistant to above treatment, refer to hospital for consideration of PUVA (psoralens and ultraviolet A radiation), methotrexate, acetretin or cyclosporin therapy.

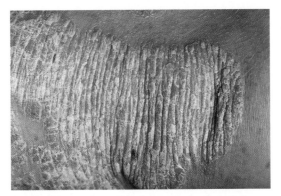

Fig. 137 Close-up of a psoriatic plaque, showing the typical silvery scales.

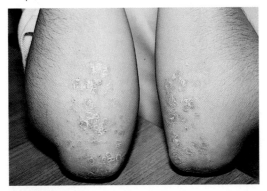

Fig. 138 Psoriasis on the elbows.

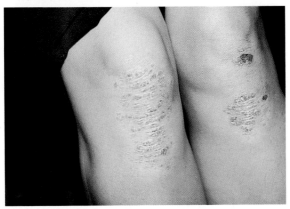

Fig. 139 Psoriasis on the knees.

A chronic polyarthritis that it is important to diagnose early, as considerable joint damage can occur in 18 months; prevented by early use of disease-modifying antirheumatic drugs (DMARDs).

Diagnosis

May initially present as a symmetrical joint inflammation affecting the MCP and DIP joints of hands (Fig. 140), the wrists, feet or knees. Early morning stiffness a feature. Refer early; if the joint symptoms have been present >2–3 months refer to a specialist. As disease progresses joint deformity occurs, e.g. boutonniere (Fig. 141) and swan-neck deformity (Fig. 142) of fingers. Rheumatoid nodules (Fig. 143) may be found on the arms and other systems may be involved, e.g. the eyes, cardiovascular, respiratory, neurological and dermatological systems. Investigations should include a full blood count, ESR/plasma viscosity/ C-reactive protein (raised if active disease), anti-nuclear antibodies (useful if considering other diseases) and rheumatoid factor. About 75% of chronic rheumatoid arthritis patients are rheumatoid factor-positive, but up to a half of patients may be negative at initial presentation. Presence of rheumatoid factor worsens prognosis. X-rays are normal early in the disease—the aim is to treat before erosions develop.

Management

Physiotherapy, occupational therapy, nursing care important. Drug therapy includes: (1) NSAIDs—for pain and swelling. Beware side-effects. May need to co-prescribe an acid-suppressing drug. (2) DMARDs, unlike NSAIDs, actually slow the progression of the disease. Start early but need close monitoring. Commonest used are methotrexate and sulphasalazine; others include hydroxychloroquine, penicillamine, gold, azathioprine, cyclosporin. (3) Steroids—intra-articular steroids helpful for individual joints but use of systemic steroids is a specialist decision.

Surgery may be required for specific joint problems.

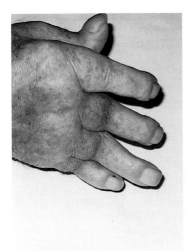

Fig. 140 The hand in severe rheumatoid arthritis: ulnar deviation, joint swelling and deformity.

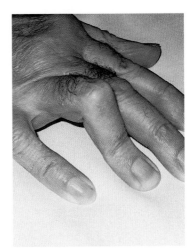

Fig. 141 The 'boutonniere' deformity, with hyperflexion at the proximal interphalangeal joint plus hyperextension at the distal interphalangeal joint.

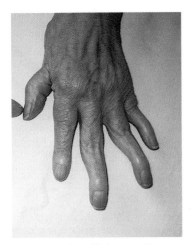

Fig. 142 A patient with 'swan neck' deformity of the fingers—note the third and fourth fingers. There is hyperextension at the proximal interphalangeal joint plus hyperflexion at the distal interphalangeal joint.

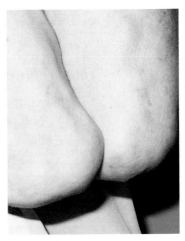

Fig. 143 Rheumatoid nodules on the arm.

Scabies

Caused by a mite. Presents as pruritis, worse at night. Red papular rash soon becomes excoriated and secondarily infected with scratching. Confirm by finding burrows, short irregular scaly lesions most frequently found between the fingers, on the wrists, abdomen, axillary folds, nipples, genitalia, ankles. Skin scrapings from burrow reveal eggs, mite faeces and mites. Spread by personal contact. Treatment: a scabicide applied to the whole body apart from the head and face. Treat all contacts. Itching may persist weeks after treatment.

Lice

Body lice in those with poor hygiene cause an itchy red rash, again commonly excoriated and secondarily infected. *Pubic lice* cause an itch and often a secondarily infected rash. Spread by sexual contact. *Head lice* (Fig. 144) cause itchy scalp but may be asymptomatic. Examine scalp, using special comb, for lice or their eggs (nits, Fig. 145). Treatment: a pediculicide, decided by a local policy. Screen all contacts, treating if infested.

Threadworms (Fig. 146)

Usually asymptomatic but can cause pruritis ani, vulvovaginitis or worms passed in the stool. Apply sticky tape to perianal skin and examine under microscope to detect ova. Treat all the family.

Verrucae (plantar warts, Fig. 147)

Usually painful, occurring on soles of foot, barely elevated from the skin with a rough hyperkeratotic appearance. If pared down there are capillary bleeding points to distinguish them from a callosity. Can resolve spontaneously. Treat with either (1) a wart preparation, paring verruca down prior to each application; or (2) cryocautery with liquid nitrogen.

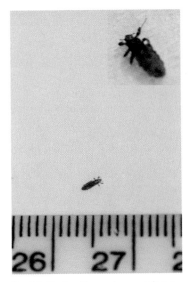

Fig. 144 The head louse shown against a centimetre rule. Inset shows magnified head louse.

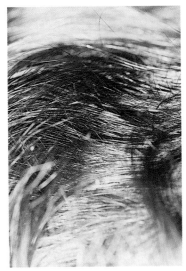

Fig. 145 'Nits'—white specks against the black hair.

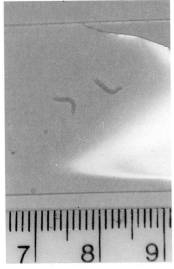

Fig. 146 Threadworms shown against a centimetre rule.

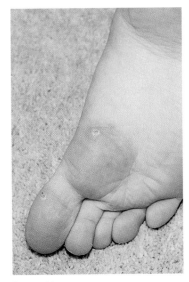

Fig. 147 Verrucae.

Causes

Arthropathies (e.g. osteoarthritis, rheumatoid arthritis, pyogenic arthritis), musculotendinous lesions (e.g. rotator cuff disorders, adhesive capsulitis, bicipital tendinitis), trauma (dislocations, fracture) and referred pain from neck (e.g. from cervical spondylosis), lung (e.g. from carcinoma bronchus), myocardium (e.g. myocardial ischaemia) and abdomen (e.g. subphrenic abscess). Elderly patients with polymyalgia rheumatica may present with shoulder stiffness.

Patient assessment

Take a history (duration, trauma, site of pain, movements that worsen the pain, other joints affected, other symptoms). Inspect the joint, palpate for tenderness, then test the full range of active and passive movement. Movements consist of abduction/adduction, flexion/extension, internal/external rotation (Figs 148–151). Always examine the cervical spine. Diagnosis made by pattern of pain, tenderness and limitation of movement, e.g. the painful arc of abduction in a rotator cuff lesion, localised tenderness of a bicipital tendinitis or the global limitation of active and passive movement with an adhesive capsulitis (frozen shoulder). The history of frozen shoulder is a 2–3 year course, starting with several months of pain, stiffness for the next 6–12 months, followed by slow (usually not complete) resolution. Common in diabetics. If all shoulder movements are normal and painless, suspect a referred cause. X-rays only helpful in excluding serious pathology. MRI scans can demonstrate rotator cuff damage.

Treatment

Depends on diagnosis. NSAIDs and physiotherapy are mainstay of treatment with steroid injections useful for a painful arc syndrome (inject the subacromial bursa), a bicipital tendinitis (do *not* inject tendon), acromioclavicular joint problems and adhesive capsulitis (inject the glenohumeral joint). Patients with a frozen shoulder may benefit from manipulation under anaesthetic. Surgery may be required for chronic rotator cuff problems, trauma or a severe arthritis.

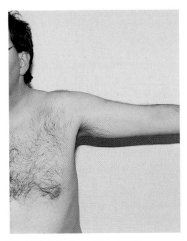

Fig. 148 Abduction of the shoulder.

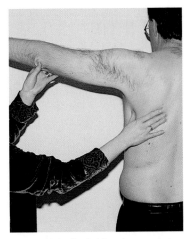

Fig. 149 Abduction holding the scapula to detect the degree of scapular movement.

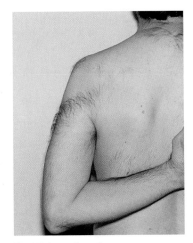

Fig. 150 Internal rotation.

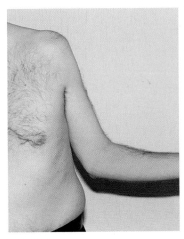

Fig. 151 External rotation.

Inflammation of the sinuses (frontal, maxillary, ethmoid). Caused by viruses or bacteria.

Diagnosis

Acute sinusitis. Presents with pain, tenderness over the affected sinus, pyrexia and a purulent or clear nasal discharge. Often follows an upper respiratory tract infection. Can cause serious complications if not adequately treated, e.g. orbital cellulitis, which needs immediate hospital admission. Other serious complications include cerebral abscess, meningitis, cavernous sinus thrombosis, osteomyelitis and mucocoele formation.

Chronic sinusitis. Presents with facial pain, tenderness over sinuses, sometimes loss of sense of smell, nasal blockage and discharge (often with postnasal drip). Pain and tenderness may be minimal or even absent. Examine nose, looking for predisposing causes, e.g. allergic rhinitis, nasal polyps, a deviated nasal septum (Fig. 152) or a past fracture. Diagnosis of sinusitis is a clinical one based on the history and examination. Plain X-rays rarely helpful (may show fluid levels in chronic sinusitis), but CT scan (Fig. 153) is investigation of choice for demonstrating sinus pathology, if required.

Treatment

Acute sinusitis. Treated with a 10-day course of a broad-spectrum antibiotic, analgesia, steam inhalation and 7 days of 1% ephedrine nose drops or use of a steroid nasal spray. The value of antibiotics has been questioned. Encourage patient to stop smoking.

Chronic sinusitis. Merits a much longer (4–8 weeks) course of antibiotics, together with a steroid nasal spray which is useful to combat any allergic component or associated nasal polyps. If no resolution of symptoms after 2 months, refer to a surgeon for further investigation and possible surgery, e.g. to reduce turbinates or correct a deviated septum.

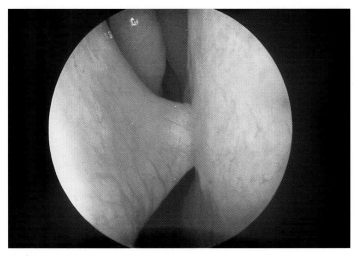

Fig. 152 Nasal septum deviated towards the left lateral nasal wall.

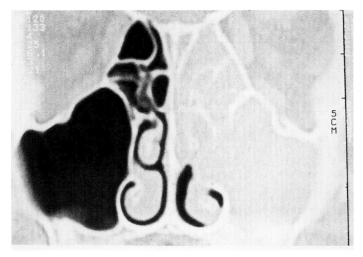

Fig. 153 A CT scan of sinuses showing 'white out' (pansinusitis) on the left.

55 / Sore throat, tonsillitis and glandular fever

Cause

Over 50% of sore throats are caused by viruses; a third are caused by *Streptococcus pyogenes* bacterium. Rare causes: blood disorders, HIV infection.

Diagnosis

Throat may be red, possibly with enlarged and/or tender cervical lymphadenopathy. Cannot guess infection from throat's appearance. Children can be more affected with systemic malaise, fever, vomiting and/or abdominal pain. Acute tonsillitis (Fig. 154) causes reddened swollen tonsils, perhaps with exudate. May be a rash with streptococcal scarlet fever. Throat swabs are of no practical value. A sore throat persisting >7 days may be due to glandular fever (GF, caused by Epstein–Barr virus). Typical features of GF (Fig. 155) include an exudative tonsillitis, palatal petechiae, cervical (possibly generalised) lymphadenopathy, enlarged spleen (in 50%), enlarged liver (in 10%) and a rash (in 10%), especially if ampicillin/amoxycillin prescribed. GF diagnosed by finding atypical lymphocytes in a full blood count and a positive Paul Bunnell/Monospot test (negative in 10% of GF patients—may take 3 weeks to turn positive). GF usually lasts 2–3 weeks in the acute stage but may be followed by weeks/months of fatigue.

Management

Antibiotic prescription rarely justified except for those with fever, exudate and glands (when streptococci commoner)—symptoms are reduced only marginally (by 12–48 h) by prescription. Antibiotics can cause allergic reactions and encourage patients to reattend for sore throats in future. Antibiotic of choice is currently penicillin for 10 days or erythromycin if sensitive. Treatment of glandular fever is symptomatic. Refer for tonsillectomy patients with recurrent tonsillitis (e.g. >5 attacks a year), unilateral tonsillar hypertrophy, quinsy or tonsils big enough to result in sleep apnoea.

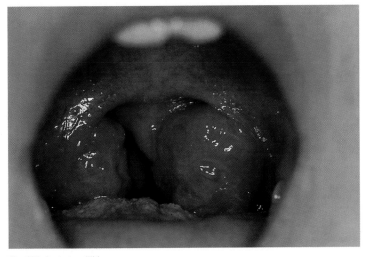

Fig. 154 Acute tonsillitis.

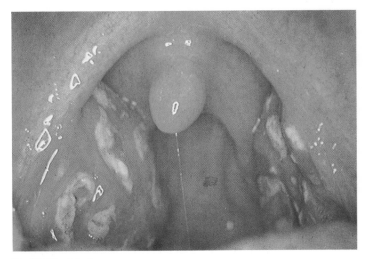

Fig. 155 Glandular fever.

Sprained ankle

Patient presents after an injury/fall with pain and/or swelling of ankle. Distinguish simple sprains from complete tears of the lateral ligament or fractures. Take history—mode of injury (inversion/twist), when swelling/bruising occurred (immediately or hours later), local tenderness, ability to bear weight. Examine to document swelling (Fig. 156), bruising (if severe, suggests a complete lateral ligament tear), local tenderness, any deformity, range of movement, stability. Also examine the Achilles tendon (? tendinitis/rupture). X-rays are indicated if (1) the patient cannot bear weight; (2) there is severe swelling/pain/bruising; (3) there is deformity, instability, excessive movement or marked bone tenderness; (4) there is no response to treatment. Simple sprains have little swelling, minimal tenderness and no bruising or instability.

Simple sprains managed immediately using ice pack, compression, elevation. A Tubigrip bandage provides support (Fig. 157) and NSAIDs are prescribed to reduce pain/swelling. Modern management is by early mobilisation with physiotherapy. Severe sprains are managed in casualty following X-ray. Application of plaster is rarely required. In a few cases of major tears of the lateral ligament with resulting instability, surgery may need to be considered.

Tennis elbow

Common condition resulting from excessive forearm use. Pain and tenderness localised to the lateral epicondyle at the site of common extensor origin. There is pain on resisted dorsiflexion of the wrist with elbow straight and forearm pronated. There is full range of movement and X-ray not required. Treat with rest and steroid injection into the area of maximum tenderness (Fig. 158). Physiotherapy helps, with surgery a final option.

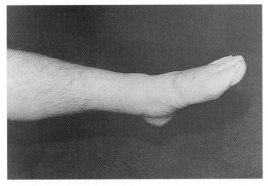

Fig. 156 A swollen sprained ankle.

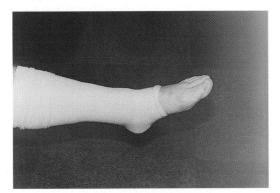

Fig. 157 A sprained ankle in a tubigrip bandage.

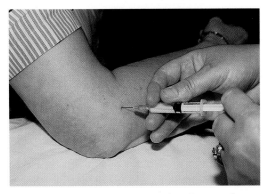

Fig. 158 Injecting steroid into the area of maximum tenderness in a tennis elbow.

WHO definition of stroke: rapidly developing clinical signs of focal (or global) disturbance of cerebral function, with symptoms lasting 24 h or longer or leading to death with no apparent cause other than of vascular origin. A TIA is an acute focal neurological deficit resolving within 24 h.

Diagnosis and investigation

Symptoms/signs depend on brain area involved. Major cerebral infarcts cause contralateral hemiplegia, dysphasia, loss of sensation, hemianopia. Bell's palsy (Fig. 159) is a differential diagnosis. Perform a neurological examination and look for hypertension, ischaemic and/or valvular heart disease, atrial fibrillation, a carotid bruit. Other risk factors include smoking, excess alcohol, polycythaemia, diabetes, hyperlipidaemia. Investigations: ESR/plasma viscosity, full blood count, urea and electrolytes, serum lipids, random blood sugar, ECG.

Management

Stroke. Refer acute strokes (within 72 h), severe headache, deteriorating conscious level, a coagulation problem, rapidly deteriorating signs, unusual symptoms/signs, uncertain diagnosis, younger patients, patients living without support. In acute ischaemic stroke, aspirin (150–300 mg/day) reduces stroke mortality and newer thrombolytic therapy in the first 3 h improves outcome. For both, need CT scan (Fig. 160) to ensure no haemorrhage. Long-term management: nursing, physiotherapy, occupational therapy, speech therapy and prevention as for TIA.

TIA. Admit if major cardiovascular problems/hypertension or multiple. Refer most for investigation, e.g. CT scan, duplex carotid scan (Fig. 161), echocardiogram. Treat risk factors, e.g. smoking, hypertension, hyperlipidaemia and atrial fibrillation. Prescribe aspirin daily (better results if combined with dipyridamole), warfarin for atrial fibrillation. Carotid endarterectomy needed if significant (>70%) carotid artery stenosis (Fig. 162).

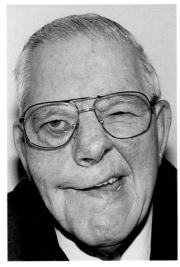

Fig. 159 Bell's palsy.

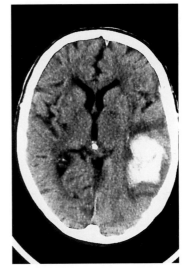

Fig. 160 Intracerebral haemorrhage on a CT scan.

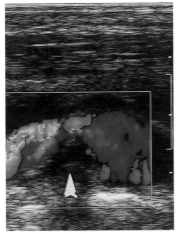

Fig. 161 Duplex scan of a carotid stenosis.

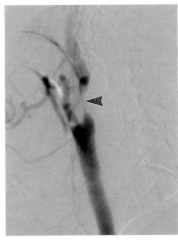

Fig. 162 Angiogram of a carotid artery stenosis.

Tinnitus

Tinnitus refers to a sensation of noise in the ears (or head), affecting about one in six adults. Commoner in elderly, often associated with hearing loss (when a hearing aid helps). Tinnitus maskers (Fig. 163) will mask the sound. Reassure patient—rare to find a major cause. Other treatments include tinnitus retraining therapy, treating anxiety/depression, counselling, relaxation techniques, acupuncture. Ménière's disease is a combination of tinnitus and/or aural fullness, recurrent rotatory vertigo and fluctuating hearing loss. In acute stage treat with vestibular sedatives; chronic disease treated with prophylactic betahistine, reduced salt intake and, in a few patients, surgery. If unilateral tinnitus or sudden onset, refer to exclude serious pathology.

Deafness

Causes

In childhood include hereditary, infection (meningitis, mumps, measles, rubella), birth trauma, otitis media with effusion. May be picked up during routine screening. *In adults* include wax, discharge, middle ear problems, otosclerosis, noise-induced, presbycusis, infection, Ménière's.

Diagnosis

Take history—speed of onset, uni/bilateral, history of infection/disease/injury, family history, job, associated symptoms, progressive or fluctuating loss. Examine for wax/discharge/perforation/signs of middle ear problems. Assess hearing (testing air and bone conduction to distinguish conductive from sensorineural deafness). Refer acute-onset deafness urgently and unilateral deafness to exclude an acoustic neuroma.

Management

Ranges from local removal of wax/discharge to surgery (e.g. stapedectomy for presbycusis) to supplying a hearing aid (Fig. 164), especially for age-related sensorineural loss of presbycusis, to insertion of a cochlear implant.

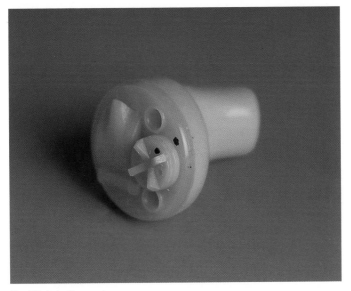

Fig. 163 A tinnitus masker.

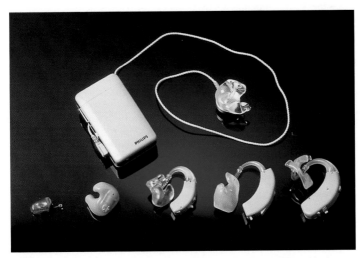

Fig. 164 A selection of hearing aids: in the ear (ITE), behind the ear (BE) and body worn (BW).

Causes	Physiological (excess normal secretions, cervical ectopy, pregnancy, the pill), infection (bacterial vaginosis (BV), *Candida*, *Trichomonas*), cervicitis (chlamydial, gonococcal, herpetic), cervical polyp, foreign body, carcinoma cervix.
Diagnosis	Take history—colour, consistency, itch, local discomfort/pain, odour, pelvic pain, last menstrual period, intermenstrual bleeding, previous infections, symptoms in contacts (? sexually transmitted disease, STD). Examine with speculum, perform a pelvic examination if appropriate and take swabs (Fig. 165); high vaginal swab useful for BV, *Candida*, *Trichomonas*, but *Gonococcus* and *Chlamydia* need endocervical swabs. *Chlamydia* is often asymptomatic but can cause pelvic inflammatory disease—a urine screening test available. Suspected STD: full testing/contact trace.
Treatment of specific infections	*Candidiasis* (Fig. 166). Presents as creamy white, cheesy, itchy discharge. Predisposing factors are antibiotics, pregnancy, diabetes, anaemia, iron deficiency. Treat with single-dose azole vaginal pessaries or oral azoles (not in pregnancy). Most cases not sexually transmitted—in single attacks no need to treat partner. For recurrent candidiasis make sure diagnosis correct, exclude precipitants, advise against use of vaginal deodorants/bubble baths/tights and treat prophylactically monthly for 6 months (patient to keep diary to determine best time for treatment) or use prolonged therapy, e.g. single-dose pessary weekly for 4–5 weeks. *BV and* Trichomonas. Present with offensive discharges, typically yellow/greenish/purulent with *Trichomonas*, and fishy/grey/non-purulent with BV. *Trichomonas* causes vulval soreness and painful vaginitis. May be symptoms in the partner. Microscopy is helpful in diagnosis, showing clue cells with BV or the *Trichomonas* protozoan. Treatment for both is metronidazole 400 mg b.d. for 7 days (treat partner as well if *Trichomonas*). Exclude co-existing STD like gonorrhoea.

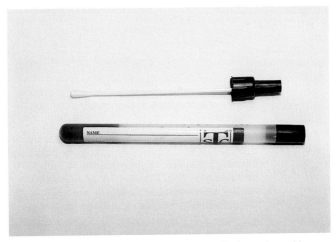

Fig. 165 Amies Charcoal Transport Swab. When investigating patients with a vaginal discharge, ensure you take the right swabs from the right sites and transport to the hospital without delay.

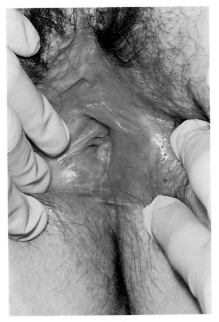

Fig. 166 Vaginal candidiasis.

Vertigo is a subjective sensation of movement when none has occurred—rotational or non-rotational.

Causes

Main causes are labyrinthitis, benign positional paroxysmal vertigo (BPPV), vestibular neuronitis, Ménière's disease, cholesteatoma, lateral semicircular canal fistula, migraine, vertebrobasilar insufficiency, multiple sclerosis, brain stem/cerebellar lesions including tumours.

Diagnosis

Take history—recent viral illness, length of symptoms, duration of an attack, associated nausea/vomiting/tinnitus/deafness, ear discharge, headache, visual disturbance, recurrence of attacks, loss of consciousness, other neurological symptoms. With BPPV, vertigo worse with the neck extended and turned to the affected side—ask specifically re. symptoms turning over in bed or on sitting up (both present in BPPV).

Examine ears (otoscopy, whispered voice and tuning fork tests), test for nystagmus and undertake a neurological examination if suggested by history. Test gait, balance (e.g. ability to stand with feet together and eyes closed) and for BPPV use the Dix–Hallpike test (Fig. 167)—vertigo and nystagmus result if BPPV is present.

Management

In family practice most cases of vertigo are due to labyrinthitis and resolve within 3–4 weeks. A vestibular sedative such as prochlorperazine or cinnarizine may help in the acute phase. BPPV is the other most common cause and may occur in clusters, lasting months or even years. Treatment of BPPV is by a series of canalolith positioning manoeuvres (e.g. Epley manoeuvre, Figs 168–170). Surgery rarely required. Treatment of other causes depends on the diagnosis. Patients with vertigo not improving after a month or with recurrent disabling attacks should be referred to a specialist.

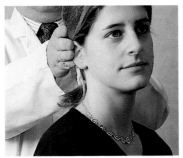
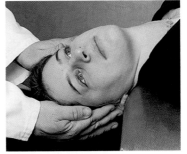

A   B

Fig. 167 Dix–Hallpike test. (A) Patient seated on couch with head turned 45° towards affected ear. (B) Patient reclines with head remaining at 45° to the affected side and 30° below the horizontal plane. Down-beating nystagmus seen.

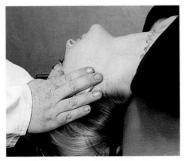
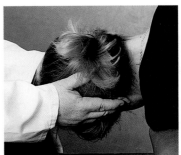

Fig. 168 An Epley manoeuvre. This comprises the first two stages as in Fig. 167, followed by turning of the head through 90° towards the unaffected ear so it lies again 45° to the vertical plane but to the opposite side.

Fig. 169 Patient turned to unaffected side with head at 45° to the vertical plane. Ensure vault of skull is directed towards the ground.

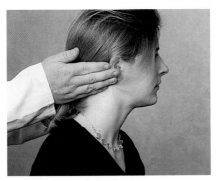

Fig. 170 Patient sits up with the head still turned towards the unaffected side.

Index